Women's Minds, Women's Bodies

Women's Minds, Women's Bodies

Interdisciplinary Approaches to Women's Health

edited by

Gwyneth Boswell
Professor of Criminology and Criminal Justice
De Montfort University

and

Fiona Poland
Director of Therapy Research
School of Occupational Therapy and Physiotherapy
University of East Anglia

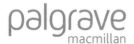

First published 2003 by
PALGRAVE MACMILLAN
Houndmills, Basingstoke, Hampshire RG21 6XS and
175 Fifth Avenue, New York, N. Y. 10010
Companies and representatives throughout the world

PALGRAVE MACMILLAN is the global academic imprint of the Palgrave
Macmillan division of St Martin's Press, LLC and of Palgrave Macmillan Ltd.
Macmillan® is a registered trademark in the United States, United Kingdom
and other countries. Palgrave is a registered trademark in the European
Union and other countries.

ISBN 0–333–91969–6

This book is printed on paper suitable for recycling and made from fully
managed and sustained forest sources.

A catalogue record for this book is available from the British Library.

Library of Congress Cataloging-in-Publication Data

Boswell, Gwyneth.
  Women's minds, women's bodies: an interdisciplinary approach to
women's health/Gwyneth Boswell, Fiona Poland.
     p. cm.
  Includes bibliographical references and index.
  ISBN 0–333–91969–6 (cloth)
  1. Women–Health and hygiene. I. Boswell, Gwyneth. II. Title.

RA778 .P724 2002
613'.042–dc21
                                                            2002026756

10 9 8 7 6 5 4 3 2 1
12 11 10 09 08 07 06 05 04 03

Printed and bound in Great Britain by
Antony Rowe Ltd, Chippenham and Eastbourne

For Janet and Monica

Contents

List of Tables and Figures

Acknowledgements

Many people have contributed to the successful completion of this book. Jenny Routledge initiated the cross-school Women's Health Initiative at the University of East Anglia, whose members undertook the stimulating discussions, activities and conferences which led to most of the chapters herein. Robbie Meehan provided excellent support for those activities, so that they were always well run and recorded; her co-ordination was essential in getting the book underway. Both Jo Campling, as commissioning editor, and the book's external reader have provided us with invaluable encouragement and advice. We are most grateful to Dan Rashid for his work in correcting many of the errors in the text that escaped us. We owe particular thanks to Jane Strudwick for her unflagging care and commitment throughout this venture, for her assiduous typing and checking of the many versions, and for keeping in touch with all those involved in this process.

Notes on the Contributors

Sara Arber, Professor and Head of Sociology Department, University of Surrey, is co-director of the University's Centre for Research on Ageing and Gender (CRAG). She was President of the British Sociological Association 1999–2001 and is well known for her work on gender and class inequalities in health, and on ageing and gender.

Gwyneth Boswell, Professor, Community and Criminal Justice Studies Unit, De Montfort University and Honorary Senior Lecturer in the Schools of Health, University of East Anglia, is a founder member of the cross-schools Women's Health Initiative at the University of East Anglia, where she was Senior Lecturer in the School of Social Work until 1998. Since then, she has worked as Principal Lecturer in Community and Criminal Justice at De Montfort University. She holds an MA and PhD and is the author of numerous research-based articles and several books, the most recent being *Imprisoned Fathers and their Children* (with Peter Wedge, 2002) based on a major research report for the Department of Health.

Joan Busfield, Professor, Department of Sociology, University of Essex, trained initially as a clinical psychologist at the Tavistock Clinic. She then worked on a study of the social influences on family size published as *Thinking about Children: Sociology and Fertility in Post-War England* (with M. Paddon, 1977). Since then her research has focused on psychiatry, gender and mental disorder and the health services. Her main publications include: *Managing Madness: Changing Ideas and Practice* (1986), *Men, Women and Madness* (1996) and *Health and Health Care in Modern Britain* (2000). She edited a special issue of the journal *Sociology of Health and Illness*, published in October 2000 as *Rethinking the Sociology of Mental Health*.

Helen Cooper, Senior Methodologist, Office for National Statistics, is helping to develop a National Statistics protocol on data sharing and confidentiality. Her research interests centre on social inequalities in health, associated with gender and ethnicity, on which she is completing a PhD.

Rosie Doy, Lecturer, Primary Care and Mental Health Nursing, School of Nursing and Midwifery, UEA, is a feminist, and has worked with women in both general hospital and community mental health and primary care settings and organisations. Her research and teaching interests include women and mental health, gender in/and health care, and supervision and support of nurses and other health care providers. She works in partnership with many professionals and standpoints and is committed to multi-professional and collaborative working.

Anne Greig, Educational Psychologist, Argyll and Bute Psychological Services Council, is a qualified and experienced teacher at pre-school, primary and A-level stages. Her research includes a PhD in development psychology (Cambridge University) and the impact of maternal depression and attachment on the social understanding of pre-schoolers (UEA). In her current role as an educational psychologist she is applying research to practice issues.

Dawn Gregory, Service and Development Manager (Child Mental Health), Norfolk Social Services Department, is a qualified nurse (1974) and social worker (1990). She has a wide range of professional and managerial experience in clinical and social care settings. Postgraduate research (1995) into the impact of parental mental illness on child development and how services are provided in this field, led to further involvement in training programmes and inter-agency protocols. Dawn is a regular contributor to child and maternal mental health conferences.

Victoria Harris, Lecturer, School of Social Work, University of East Anglia, teaches on the MA/Dip. in Social Work and is also Director of the East Anglian Practice Teaching Programme for qualified social workers. She is a former Senior Probation Officer with particular experience of working with women's groups. She has written about adolescent sex offenders and is currently evaluator for the Norfolk Youth Offending Teams.

Barbara Hewson, Barrister, Littman Chambers, was called to the Bar of England and Wales in 1985, and to the Bar of Ireland in 1991. She was the first recipient of the *Lawyer Magazine's* 'Barrister of the Year' award in 1998. She was Junior Counsel for Ms. S. in the St George's case.

Jan Keene, Professor of Primary Care, Department of Health and Social Care, University of Reading, has carried out research in the drug and alcohol field for 20 years, publishing four books and 26 papers in refereed journals.

Catherine Locke, Lecturer in Development Studies, School of Development Studies, University of East Anglia, Norwich, holds a doctorate and has a background in social development and gender relations. Her past work on reproduction has focused on the relationship between gender and fertility, and the quality of family planning care in India and Kenya. She is currently working on the way in which different institutions have interpreted, advocated and implemented rights-based approaches to reproduction in diverse contexts.

Alison Macfarlane is Professor of Perinatal Health, Department of Midwifery, St Bartholomew School of Nursing and Midwifery, City University. After studying mathematics at Oxford and statistics at University College, London, Alison worked as a statistician in agricultural research, and on transportation studies, and was a programmer in automated cartography before becoming a medical statistician. After working at the MRC Air Pollution Unit and London School of Hygiene and Tropical Medicine, she was employed for 23 years at the National Perinatal Epidemiology Unit, until leaving in 2001 to move to City University.

Judy Moore, Director of Counselling, University of East Anglia, has worked within the person-centred approach for counselling since the mid-1980s, and has taught for several years on the Diploma in Counselling at the University of East Anglia, where she is also a part-time lecturer in the School of Education and Professional Development.

Miranda Mugford, Professor of Health Economics, School of Medicine, Health Policy and Practice, University of East Anglia, is co-ordinator of a growing health economics group at UEA. Until 1997, she was an economist at the National Perinatal Epidemiology Unit in Oxford. Since moving to UEA she has continued her work on perinatal health services, including the two-volume book *Birth Counts* (co-authored with Alison Macfarlane).

Christine Nightingale, Senior Lecturer in Health Studies, De Montfort University, began her career as a nurse and a teacher for people with learning disabilities. Her recognition of the health inequalities of vulnerable groups led her to undertake PhD research, exploring health policy and barriers to health care access, with particular reference to cervical screening. She is currently researching the impact of learning on health.

Gillian Oaker, Clinical Psychologist, Norfolk Mental Health Care Trust, qualified as a clinical psychologist in 1988 from the University of Leicester. She has since worked exclusively within the NHS in adult mental health. Women's health has been the focus of the majority of her clinical and academic work. After completing cognitive behaviour therapy training at Oxford she has continued to use this approach with many adults who are referred to the NHS.

Fiona Poland, Director of Therapy Research, School of Occupational Therapy and Physiotherapy, University of East Anglia, is a member of the cross-schools Women's Health Initiative at the University of East Anglia. She holds a PhD and is author of *Sociology in Practice for Health Care Professionals* (with Ron Iphofen, 1999).

Roberta Sassatelli, Lecturer in Sociology, School of Economic and Social Studies, University of East Anglia, holds an MA and PhD, and teaches sociology at the University of East Anglia. She has published widely on social and cultural theory, consumer organizations, consumer culture, fitness culture, gender and the body. She is author of *Anatomia della Palestra, il Mulino* (2000). She is currently completing a monograph on contemporary consumer practices.

Wendy Savage, Honorary Professor Middlesex University, Dept. of Social Service, Medical School of St Bartholomew's and Royal London Queen Mary University of London, qualified as a doctor in 1960, from Cambridge University and London Hospital Medical College. She has worked in the USA, Nigeria, Kenya and New Zealand. She returned to the UK and was appointed Senior Lecturer in Obstetrics and Gynaecology in 1977. Since this time she has also been Press Officer for 'Doctors for a Woman's Choice in Abortion'. She is a supporter of natural childbirth, and came to prominence when she was unjustly suspended and then reinstated in 1985–6.

Introduction: Exploring Women's Health – Differences, Discourses and Disciplines

Gwyneth Boswell and Fiona Poland

So we can see that gender inequalities in access to a wide range of resources have a significant impact on the health of women. Though they have a longer average life expectancy than men, they do not necessarily lead healthier lives. And most importantly, a considerable amount of the illness they experience can be traced back in one way or another to the nature of their daily lives and should therefore be preventable through public policy.

(Doyal, 2000: p. 939)

While many women, especially in the developed world, are living longer, reviews of recent research, notably that of the World Health Organization's Gender and Health Working Group (Doyal et al., 1998), have clearly demonstrated how women are subject to health inequalities conditioned by wider socio-economic inequalities: mental stress and poverty linked to their care roles (Barnett and Marshall, 1991; Bartley et al., 1992; Belle, 1990); restricted access to health services or to health policy decision-making (Brems and Griffiths, 1993; Doyal, 1985; Gijsbers van Wijk et al., 1996; Standing, 1997; Timyan et al., 1993); health problems relating to reproductive systems (Germain et al., 1992) and women's preponderance in the ageing population (WHO, 1996). Enabling women's health, therefore, raises multi-layered issues which cannot be solved simply by focusing on the individualized interventions which characterize a purely medical approach. What is also required is a means to understand and act on the multifactorial context which influences the health of women's minds and bodies.

Health researchers such as Bird and Rieker (1999) have argued strongly that an integrated approach is needed to build effective health

1

care which recognizes the complex nature of differences in men's and women's health. These are not only biological, but also relate to different patterns of actions and experiences in their everyday lives. Such gendered differences have been overlooked in the design of clinical studies for many reasons (DeBruin, 1994; Rosser, 1994). Ethnic dimensions have been similarly neglected. The wide range of health and social care value bases which lie at the heart of professional responses to women's health issues have tended to be more implicit than explicit. An interdisciplinary approach, which brings together branches of learning, can help both lay and professional decision-making. Crucial here is building an understanding of when to attend to individuals' health behaviours, concerns and access to care and when to work for policies which address the impact of social, economic or other factors on the health of women who also may be members of disadvantaged groups. Such an approach is essential if we are to understand influences on women's ability actively to tackle and address health risks.

In 1997 a group of women staff, from a range of schools at the University of East Anglia, came together to form a Women's Health Initiative to work across academic disciplines to examine working issues in women's health. The discussions that followed emphasized the complexity of links between women's physical and mental health and how these may be understood and experienced both positively and negatively. The activities of this group drew on current perspectives from a range of disciplines. Some of these disciplines were directly concerned with the professional provision of health care, such as clinical psychology, nursing, medicine, counselling and social work; some related to professions often interacting with health services, such as social work and law; and some were disciplines that can be used to study health issues, such as history, sociology, economics and criminology. Research reports from each of these disciplines provided telling images and experiences of how women's health issues can often be treated with ambivalence. It became clear that developing insights across such different disciplines can also help generate alternative methodologies, discourses and resources to provide sounder evidence for engaging with women's health issues. The work presented in this book draws on different approaches brought together through the group's activities.

Much of the research and practice described relates to women's health in the context of the 'developed' Western world. However, this introductory chapter makes a point of chronicling a range of research findings in respect of women in the developing world. This is in order to set the topic of interdisciplinary women's health in a global context and to highlight the added dimensions for health and well-being of those individuals and groups who are both female and of differing cultural and ethnic origins from the majority of women described in the ensuing chapters. For all, the confluence of inter-disciplinarity can help point to the elements and uses of a more holistic analytical framework within which to encourage appropriate and empowering dialogues for evaluating women's health options, wherever they are in the world.

Historical, social and psychoanalytic methods can be used dynami-cally to engage with images of women's health. The values placed on the health of women by themselves, and by groups in which they live, are developed over time and in the context of interaction and reflection. Women's attitudes and actions to their own bodies may encompass the expression of self-appreciation or of self-hatred. Experiences of abuse may be reflected in diverse physical and mental expressions of their state of ill- or well-being. The possibilities for women to play an active and empowered role in building their own health may be constructed in varyingly positive or negative ways within the diverse discourses of families, professions and institutions. Viewing women's health from an international perspective highlights the existence of contrasting and unequal constraints on women's expe-rienced choices, related stresses and, consequently, on their options for action. Women cannot be seen simply as victims of illness or events, or passive recipients of health care and health policies, when their collec-tive and individual efforts are often central to the provision of health care and to the formulation of the policies themselves.

Women's interaction with health services and policy can and should constitute the bridge between the health of individuals and the response of communities and wider society. The degree of strength of this interface may well make the difference to women's minds and bodies being built or broken. Particularly significant here are the dimensions of risk to health and well-being which are posed, not only by the individual actions of women themselves, but by the cultural and structural frameworks which provide the context of events, under-standings and actions.

Active decision-making processes are conditioned by constraining structures exemplified in public policy-making as it is reflected in legis-lation. So, for instance, in the field of mental health, reactive processes can be discerned, which formalize not only legislation itself, but also within it the values, norms, attitudes and beliefs of society which are prevalent at any given time. This encompasses stereotyping processes which may construct women as victims who have emotional or psychological problems: 'woman as provocateuse', 'woman as property', 'woman as hysteric', 'woman as liar', and so on (Salasin and Rich, 1993: 947). Women need to be fully aware of these social constructs in order to combat them, and to be proactive in redefining them to fill the gap between real needs and policy response. Such informed action is a positive alternative to the guilt and self-blame to which women are traditionally prone, and which often leads them into further situations of powerlessness, such as involvement in abusive relationships (Carmen and Rieker, 1989). Enacting this alternative engages the woman in maturation, strengthened self-belief and the ability to identify and then reject inadequate stereotypes (Burt and Katz, 1987). Such active decision-making can foster a sense of mission to take responsibility for contributing to change.

This project none the less engages women in the arena of risk-taking and, therefore, also calls for informed risk management. For the purposes of this publication, Kemshall's definition of risk will be taken – 'the probability that an event or behaviour carrying the possibility of an adverse or negative outcome will occur' (Kemshall, 1998: p. 4). There are multiple hazards in proactivity as well as in passivity, which need to be considered, analysed and comparatively weighed, and this is where the knowledge and perspectives generated by a range of disciplines may well be relevant. Whether women remain in the culturally prescribed roles often imposed on them by the health framework, or whether they consciously choose to break out of these roles, they are located along a continuum of risk. As a UK ministerial publication notes: 'the government recognises that poor people, particularly women, are the most vulnerable to all forms of crime and civil conflict, including domestic violence, and that in very many cases, formal justice systems fail to protect them' (DFID, 2000: p. 2). For centuries, and across the world, they have been the victims of the majority of domestic violence and child abuse (including child prostitution) and, in the United States, for example, are alleged to be at greater risk of violent crime than of breast cancer, other cancers, high blood pressure and other well-known health problems (Koss, 1990; Salasin and Rich, 1993). By virtue of their gender, and without taking action on their own account, they are thus propelled onto the risk continuum. Once on it, they are liable to move along the path to further victimization, self-harm and even, in some cases, to anti-social or criminal behaviour, wherein the link between home violence, street survival and street crime still goes unrecognized (Chesney-Lind, 1997). This is despite the fact that many women serving prison sentences are known to be the victims of abuse (Boswell, 1996; HM Inspectorate of Prisons, 1997).

Women frequently reach the high risk end of the continuum via a wide range of physical and mental health problems associated with the above types of progression (Campbell, 1995; Plichta, 1996). Corbin et al. (2001), for example, show how college women with severe victimization histories, compared with non-victims, reported more consensual sexual partners, less perceived assertiveness in ability to refuse unwanted sexual advances, greater weekly alcohol consumption and more positive outcome expectancies for alcohol, including tension reduction, sexual enhancement and global positive change. As the authors point out, such self-treatment places them at high risk of sexual violence:

> Men's attributions with regard to women's alcohol consumption, coupled with the resulting impairment in women's perception of risk as well as their less assertive sexual behaviour, create a potentially dangerous synergy of risk factors for these women. (Corbin et al., 2001: p. 307)

This is not to suggest as the broad solution to avoiding male predators that previously victimized women should drink less alcohol, since this would return women to their stereotypic label as provocateuse. However, if they were provided both with the knowledge that increased alcohol intake raised their risk of exposure to further violence, together with some techniques of resistance to such attacks (whether verbal or physical) this would, at the very least, improve their capacity to choose in respect of alcohol consumption (Norris et al., 1996).

Similarly, longitudinal research on women's responses to relationship battering has described a process whereby most women choose to adopt a set of responses to achieve non-violence via both physical and mental leaving and returning (Campbell et al., 1998). They described responding to turning points by thinking about, labelling and conceptualizing what was happening to them; by negotiating internally with themselves and externally with the abuser; and by experimenting with strategies to improve the relationship and decrease the abuse. This research countered popular notions of the 'passive' victim and revealed active decision-making processes which needed to be supported by advocacy and partnership for the women's goal of staying safe, and therefore healthy, to be achieved.

Such active assessment and management of these points of risk are crucial, since known health problems accruing to women who sustain long-term physical abuse include: physical injury requiring hospital treatment; chronic pain; headaches; neurological problems; irritable bowel syndrome; digestive problems; eating disorders; pelvic inflammatory disease; sexually transmitted diseases, including HIV and AIDS; vaginal and anal tearing; bladder infections; sexual dysfunction; pelvic pain; urinary tract infections; unintended pregnancy; and varying degrees of depression (Campbell and Socken, 1999; Heise et al., 1995).

These comparative risks of passivity and proactivity in adverse circumstances are not always, however, easy to assess, especially at crisis points. Thus, it is essential that means are available to consider, analyse and weigh them so that the chosen response is not one which sets off a further chain of harm to the woman's physical and mental health. However, there are other kinds of risks which often do not come accompanied by any real possibility of choice. These are contexts of risk which obtain simply by virtue of where women live across the world, the cultural and religious practices in which they participate, willingly or otherwise, and their levels of access to resources in the surrounding region, such as transport. Seen from an international perspective, comparative risks to women's health multiply. Whereas in the UK, one in 5,000 pregnancies results in a woman's death, in the poorest countries, such as Sierra Leone, the figure is one in seven. Their chances of survival are directly linked to access to basic health care. It is not always the complete absence of such a health care facility that is the problem, but rather the lack of any kind of transport by which to reach it (Thaddeus and Maine, 1991). Simple provision of transport can thus significantly reduce health risk and, thereby, increase both choice and independence.

A notable example of a cultural practice which heightens risks for women in terms of sexual health, in childbirth and beyond, is that of female genital mutilation. Despite being illegal in very many countries, it continues to be carried out in parts of Asia, Africa, the Arabian Peninsula and within some immigrant populations in the Western world. Apart from the immediate health consequences of this damaging practice, when infibulation is part of the mutilation process, it frequently causes acute complications and pain in childbirth (Toubia and Izett, 1998). In some cases, this practice is perpetrated on quite young women, especially where their culture advocates early marriage. Early marriage, in its turn, often prevents young women from completing primary education if they are removed from school on marriage, or expelled if they become pregnant (Bureau of International Labor Affairs, 1998). Other young women may be kept away from school because of child and adolescent labour practices, including domestic slavery and the sex industry. These often result in low school enrolment, high absentee and drop-out rates attributable to fatigue from long hours of labour, work-related injuries and illnesses. Young women, in fact, constitute two-thirds of all children not attending school in the developing world, notably in predominantly rural areas (Bureau of International Labor Affairs, 1998). This greatly reduces their access to literacy and an awareness of their legal and human rights – both highly relevant to their mental and physical health chances. Their lack of education deprives them of fundamental life-skills and knowledge which would otherwise afford them protection from risk and increase awareness and choice about their way of life (Bureau of International Labor Affairs, 1996, 1998).

Cultural values clearly impinge on the level of risks women encounter in the increasingly important sphere of HIV/AIDS prevention and care (Weeks et al., 1996). Some traditional beliefs include those of witchcraft, which may construct the notion that HIV/AIDS is a punishment for infidelity. Bearing in mind the social constructs referred to earlier, women are obvious targets here. In sub-Saharan Africa, where over two-thirds of the world's HIV/AIDS population reside, young women are disproportionately affected (UNAIDS/WHO, 1998). Up to eight times more adolescent girls than boys are living with the disease. Girls are more susceptible to infection because of the tearing of the hymen at first intercourse, and because immature vaginal walls are easily damaged. Their low social status and bargaining power and their need for economic support also place them at risk. Some healing traditions in Africa suggest that sex with a virgin girl will cure HIV/AIDS (CIIR, 1999). Thus, the health risks to young women of contracting a disease which may kill eventually are very considerable in these societies.

Rape victims of all ages are also at high risk because of the bleeding and consequent potential HIV transmission which may result from violation. In health care terms, women giving birth to babies to whom they have transmitted the disease may find that any available medical attention is given to the child, rather than to them (CIIR, 1999). The long-term problem here is that the child's capacity to thrive may well depend on the survival of its mother. Thus, the health risk to both mother and child is increased by this short-sighted and resource-inefficient practice. Such cultural biases feed into the broader issue of prevention and treatment programmes in mother-child transmission.

A child can become infected with HIV pre-natally, at the time of delivery or post-natally through breast-feeding. Infection at delivery is the most common, leading to the practice of Caesarean section (with its own attendant hazards, as Savage shows in Chapter 7) as a method of reducing the risk of HIV infection (Whiteside and Sunter, 2000). However, much research has been carried out into the use of anti-retroviral drugs which may inhibit viral reproduction in the infant. The administration of the drug AZT to HIV-positive pregnant women has shown transition reduction rates of between 37 and 67.5 per cent (Gray, 1998). Nevertheless, its cost and the complexity of ensuring patients' adherence to it have meant that, until early 2001, only mainly wealthy nations were able to make use of it. With the recent relenting of drug companies in respect of drug costs to developing countries, it is to be hoped that transmission prevention can now begin in earnest. The extent to which this reduces the actual risk to pregnant mothers of developing AIDS remains to be seen. However, such provision should significantly reduce the likelihood of societies and individual mothers having to expend scarce health resources on caring for a sick child. If other prevention programmes operate effectively during their children's lifetime, such transmission prevention should also reduce the longer-term health risks for their own daughters. The success of this combination of knowledge and social and economic action has, at least, created a zone of hope for future risk limitation.

In the meantime, many other types of risk obtain for women living in the harshly poor, usually rural environments of the developing world. Not only are their children obliged to labour, but the adult women frequently bear the main burden of responsibility for basic family survival (Boserup, 1970). Despite, being regarded in many cultures as unclean and generally inferior, they nevertheless grow the food, fetch the water and fuel (frequently from miles away) and do the marketing, as well as rearing the children (Moore, 1988). Often this is exacerbated by the men of the family migrating to urban areas to seek employment; often too, these men do not return. As one author has noted, 'In parts of sub-Saharan Africa as many as 70 per cent of rural households are headed by women. The physical and emotional wear hardly needs description' (Elliott, 1988: p. 27).

The fact that two-thirds of the world's population still live in absolute poverty means that the majority of the world's women lack the basic necessities of human existence (UN, 1995). As such, their life expectancy, infant mortality rate, nutrition levels, literacy, access to health care and much more are significantly less than those of women in the Western world (Sen, 1988). Not only are these risks physical, there are also risks to the psyche: fear, anxiety, insecurity, superstition, loneliness, despair, anger, the effects of discrimination, and so on (for example, Desjarlais et al., 1995; Reichenheim and Harpham, 1991). No figures can adequately capture their scope but, as contributors such as Doy, Keene and Oaker show in chapters 3, 4 and 9 respectively, such psychological stresses are frequently inimical to women's health and well-being. Any chance of reducing this combination of risks to women's minds and bodies rests on a huge complexity of potential change agents. The rural poverty cycle develops from high birth-rates, increasing pressure from both larger human and animal populations, deforestation, erosion, competition for land, lower rainfall, lower soil fertility, poor grazing, cattle failing to thrive and thus insufficient food for the surrounding population. Wholesale global remedies are needed to change this state of affairs. Aid programmes, the setting of international prices, reduction of trade barriers, cancellation of debt, increased availability of medical and other technology are all factors which, given the international will, would reduce the risks to women and children (WHO, 1995).

However, simply to relate such health risks to women is to engender a counsel of despair. That women have been, are and are likely to continue to be vulnerable and victimized by reason of their sex is indisputable. That such risks vary hugely according to their geographical location in the world is also not a matter for debate. Global, political and legal remedies are certainly required. But women have always been innovators, practised in the art of compromise and of finding ways through barriers. In this way, they clearly challenge notions of 'victim feminism' and evince their own, usually unlabelled and unsung 'power feminism' within their personal settings. As Wolf recounts, women in America have begun defending themselves from rape with knives and firearms; in Sarajevo many reacted to rape and other forms of victimization by rejecting their submissive roles and joining the military (Wolf, 1994). More peaceful forms of proactivity are to be found in a range of other innovative ventures across the world, such as the distinctive cross-stitch embroidery co-operatives operating across Palestinian refugee camps in the West Bank (Farah, 1996).

Equally challenging issues are raised by the activities of Chinese feminists who seek to bring about a change in women's lives in relation to the 'one-child-per-family' policy in force for the last 20 years. In the face of a repressive regime, they are beginning to speak out about the impact of state birth planning on women's bodies and on their wider existence. While there is a positive side to women being able to control their child-bearing capacity, the negative side includes the risk to them from surgical procedures – intrauterine device insertion, sterilization and abortion – and the social pressure when they fail to produce a son, a preference deeply rooted in Chinese culture. The consequences have included significant levels of abandonment and infanticide of girl babies and rising rates of suicide amongst rural women who fail to produce a son (Small Group, 1999). A research study looked at how women managed to work for, and feel optimistic about, improving their reproductive health and freedom against a background of discouragement of female empowerment. This showed how they managed to advance their objectives through broadening rather than repudiating existing discourses (Greenhalgh, 2001). They introduced ideas from abroad through international conferences and seminars, and sought to expand already legitimated language emanating from such fora, as a means of gradually suggesting change in the official population control policy. One research respondent explained her strategy in terms of what, effectively, constituted a risk assessment:

> If you are too critical, or if you move too fast or just too hard, the government will close you down and deprive you of a voice. The most productive approach ... is to propose ways to help the government, offering formulas it can accept. Given the continued power of the party and the state, today one must work with the government, not against it. Tomorrow things might be different. (Greenhalgh, 2001: p. 880)

These women are able to feel positive about this subtle approach simply because their perspectives have not been officially repudiated, and this negotiation of sanction is a vital ingredient of their assessment and consequent ability to manage the risk associated with expressing their views.

Moving away from politics, however, the role that stark economic changes can play in raising, as well as more frequently diminishing, the role of women – and thus their psychological well-being – is set out in a study conducted on Indonesian women and their families (Hancock, 2001). During 1997 and 1998, the international economic 'Asian crisis' produced massive inflation and currency devaluation in Indonesia. Subsequently, young women working in factories began to contribute greater proportions of their earnings to their households and, as a consequence, their status improved. Traditional patriarchy decreased as the women's earning power enabled them to play a more central part in household decision-making. One consequence was that some young women reported with pride the fact that their earnings would help their female siblings to complete their high school educa- tion and potentially break free of the traditions of early marriage and early school-leaving referred to above. Such advances demonstrate the importance of access to resources and networks in the promotion of women's health and well-being.

The above examples show very clearly that women do not have to compound their cultural lack of power by sinking into a state of 'surplus powerlessness' (Lerner, 1991). By implicitly assessing their levels of risk and finding ways to manage these, it becomes possible for them to draw on a variety of means consciously to widen their options and actively overcome the oppressions which surround them, with major effects on their health and well-being. Paradoxically, socio- economic trends and developments in medicine and technology have helped the control of many groups of women over their health in some areas but reduced it in others (Haynes, 1991; Waldron and Jacobs, 1989). Such contradictory tendencies indicate that a more complete conceptualization of dilemmas and solutions in women's health action can be achieved only if means are found to recognize differences between women and between the sexes. It is also necessary to break down boundaries of practice and communication between women's health and their wider roles, which means drawing on an integrated, holistic framework for constructing dialogues through which to assess and manage risk.

The growing literature on risk, including risks in managing health (for example, Gabe, 1995), has underlined the need to understand the degree of ambivalence surrounding this, which can mean that definitions of risk may conflict and shift. As Scott and Freeman (1995) have stressed in the context of HIV/AIDs prevention, risk management cannot be a simple question of health professionals encouraging 'rational' risk awareness and prescribing uniform strategies of risk avoidance. Such professionals may also find themselves working in risky ways (Coleman and Dickinson, 1984) and in ways which compete with each other and with 'their' patients (Graham and Oakley, 1981; Miles, 1991). Power structures may constrain the options of many different groups of women (Holland et al., 1990). Ideal and uniform choices are clearly not available to all women in similar ways. Bloor (1995) argues for the usefulness of sociological theoretical concepts such as 'systems of relevances' (Schutz, 1970) as a way to develop a heuristic framework to deal with the diversity of risk practices. Such an approach recognizes that developing priorities and means of dealing with risks must be related to the practical realities for women of weighing their costs and benefits for their different everyday lives. The diverse expertise of women themselves, whether lay or professional, is clearly vital for determining priorities for action.

Such considerations underline the importance of examining the local and informal in greater, holistic detail if we are to understand women's position in relation to health. This is highlighted by the recent debates among policymakers and health researchers about the potential of a concept of social capital for addressing health inequalities. This follows the impact of research in political science such as that of Putnam (1993) and in health (for example, Wilkinson, 1996), which suggested that communities with higher rates of civic participation and networks based on reciprocal relationships are likely to generate better health outcomes. Yet both the specific effects on women, and their contribution to the social and health capital of communities in the face of global fragmenting influences, has been largely overlooked. This is partly because of the literature's over-concentration on more formal institutions of public participation where proportions of women, though increasing, are often small. But it is also partly because, as Lowndes (2000) notes, this research has largely overlooked the contribution of women in generating social capital through community-based activities such as voluntary work, relating to diverse forms of care, which characteristically demonstrate mutuality and reciprocity. These clearly constitute networks which help form social capital and can directly and indirectly help sustain healthy lives. Even as women are increasingly engaged in formal employment, research such as Russell's (1999) indicates that such women's involvement in care networks and neighbourliness may be more rather than less important for the effective everyday coordination of home, work and family life. An effective concept of social capital, therefore, needs to be one which redirects its attention from citizenship within formal political arenas to the 'small democracies' of everyday life networks and neighbourliness. These also indicate the multiple and conflicting agendas which individual women may be managing (Poland, 1991) and which may constrain their management of risk as indicated by Grinyer's observations on managing HIV/AIDS risks in health care occupations (Grinyer, 1995).

Ways in which women can participate in, and take control of, defining and managing the levels of risk in their lives need to be opened up for examination, as illustrated implicitly and explicitly in the chapters in this book. Women can be seen to equip themselves with knowledge and understandings of relevant historical contexts, health care policies and legislation, resources and supportive networks. All of these can be drawn on if we are to build a protective but flexible framework for health in women's everyday lives, to reduce the risks surrounding them, while also recognizing which of those risks women themselves see as important to address, and why.

In this book, diverse disciplines are drawn on to engage with a range of women's physical and mental health issues at individual, community and international levels. Disciplinary differences can be used to extend the diversity of discourses which may mediate enabling and disabling actions, knowledge and resources. Heightening awareness of risks in relation both to health enablement and disablement can be assisted by looking beyond the boundaries of one discipline to focus on problem issues which may have been overlooked, or where problem-solving actions, resources or networks may have been developed. Each chapter provides insights – some predominantly theoretical, some predominantly practice-based, most an integration of the two – into how women's health issues can be reframed within different discourses. Through them, ideas can be generated as to which problems, resources and courses of action can be defined and addressed.

Part I sets out some historical aspects of the conceptualization of women's health and of their roles in healing. Such perspectives can offer insights into patterns and images of political and cultural empowerment and subordination, in terms of both what themes may persist and what may be presented as traditional, while closer examination reveals continual changes. Harris's chapter delineates the persisting polarization of stereoptypical images of women as healers and men as doctors within enduring themes in the gender relations of health. Her exploration of how such images may have been reinforced and resisted helps provide a context for recognizing health issues and actions raised in later chapters. Sociological approaches to health have frequently been directed at cultural and professional practices which have affected women's health roles. This is exemplified by Busfield's historical sociological examination of how the establishment of psychiatric practices has not been gender-neutral. She traces the ways in which categorizations of mental illness, such as epilepsy and shell shock, and services developed to accommodate problems posed by predominantly male experiences in the late nineteenth and early twentieth centuries, but came to be assigned more frequently to women to accord with prevailing views of femininity.

Part II focuses on how women may view, describe and use their bodies in ways which may both strengthen and harm their health. Nursing perspectives help focus on issues of care management and patient support. Doy's chapter, drawing on her research with mental health nurses, points up the paradoxes in women's higher rates of bodily self-mutilation and the need to build positive discourses with such women if they are to be understood as more than victims and provided with appropriate health care which includes risk management. Much psychological research has been directed at understanding psychological abilities and attitudes and on evaluating the effectiveness of therapeutic interventions. Keene's examination of patterns of women's use and misuse of drugs and alcohol, and current psychologically informed treatments, suggests that such use appears to be subject to extremes of social sanction or encouragement, depending on the context of use. She emphasizes that social and psychological, and not only medical and psychiatric, approaches are required to support their active role in managing such risks. Moore argues for the appropriateness for women of counselling which is body-aware as well as person-centred. This is illustrated through the detailed analysis of the case history of a woman client involved in a painful and decentring family health care process. Although exercise may often be viewed as unambiguously healthy, Sassatelli's sociological examination queries how far this can be the case for women, given the cultural tensions surrounding body ideals exemplified by women's choices of gymnastic techniques such as body-building, aerobics, yoga and soft gym.

Part III recognizes that different discourses, dialogues and professional value bases may construct women's health in a variety of ways which are empowering or disempowering for women. Savage draws on her medical experience as an obstetrician to query how far consumerism and an 'information society' have really opened up the range of women's choices in childbirth. She critiques health organizational practices and policies which limit the promotion of women's childbirth choices in the modern health service. Health decisions are often linked to legal rights and responsibilities, which may be evoked to support or suppress women's health choices. From her perspective as a practising barrister, Hewson examines outcomes and women's resistance, in recent legal processes, of pressures to declare pregnant women incompetent to decide on the acceptability of levels of risk for medical interventions to be employed during labour.

The recent higher visibility of female survivors of child sexual abuse has itself posed challenges for addressing their related health problems. How mental and physical health problems relating to their abuse may be identified, and then helped, is a matter of some controversy. Drawing on her work as a clinical psychologist, Oaker overviews the usefulness of cognitive behavioural therapy strategies employed with adult women who have been sexually abused in childhood. She exemplifies this with a detailed case study of a woman's progress towards managing a range of mental health issues linked to earlier sexual abuse. Women are at greater risk of developing depression than are men but, given the prominence of women's activities in maintaining relationships, this is more than simply a problem for individual women. Greig and Gregory examine the implications of recent psychological research for postnatal depression for relationship-building, relating these to findings from two detailed case studies of maternal mental health. Nightingale's chapter draws on inclusive nursing research on the access of women with learning difficulties to cervical screening. She demonstrates how health professionals' judgements about health status and communication abilities can lead to disadvantaged groups of women being excluded from services aimed at reducing cancer risk.

Part IV highlights the examination of local and international policy-related trends and alliances which affect women's health. MacFarlane and Mugford, with backgrounds in statistics and health economics respectively, evaluate influences on trends in maternity care in the UK and the role of women in actively shaping maternity policies and services. Whilst the twentieth century clearly saw dramatic improvements in maternal and infant mortality and morbidity, there have been marked divergences between groups and generations about priorities for and means of action in this area. Women comprise the majority of older people but older women do not constitute one group. Cooper and Arber analyse UK survey statistics to underline this in relation to the little examined area of socio-economic effects on the health of older minority ethnic women. Taking the example of tobacco use, they remind us how specifically health differences may be related to differences in risk-laden cultural practices such as smoking and tobacco chewing. The issue of dealing with differences through negotiation and networking is reinforced by Locke's analysis of progress towards international agreement on a reproductive rights agenda in the face of multiple interpretations of the definition and importance of women's reproductive rights.

We have seen that a dynamic and holistic analysis of women's health issues is, therefore, required. A framework for health risk assessment for women, is one which can take account of diverse ways in which groups of women may need to equip themselves with knowledge and discourses of various kinds, as outlined through the following chapters, in ways which matter to their everyday lives. A suitable framework should, therefore, be a flexible one which can be used to re-view the subject of analysis in both positive and negative terms, as well as holistically in bodily, emotional, mental and environmental terms, with reference to a variety of dimensions and methodologies. It should, thus, facilitate dialogue across disciplines and between different groups of women, both lay and professional, to draw on and build knowledge of contexts, connections and processes for health change and action.

Much of our present discussion resonates with a range of recent explanations of health and health action. Arguing for the potential contribution of interdisciplinary approaches in addressing women's health issues certainly posits the need to look beyond the boundaries of increasingly challenged biomedical approaches. The articulation of diverse interests and perspectives has become more frequently endorsed in cultural and academic approaches such as postmodernism (e.g. Fox, 1993) and in the work of community-based movements and feminism (e.g. Doyal, 1995). Such challenges have drawn attention to the micro- and macro-political interests of those groups, including health professional groups which may assert the dominance of specific explanations of health. In contrast, empirical research on health explanations, such as that of Stainton Rogers (1991) has emphasized the fluidity and multiplicity of individuals' use in practice of not just one but multiple frameworks of health, whether in their work as health professionals or as lay members of society.

In seeking to understand health action, health promoters have increasingly drawn on approaches which take account of lay perspectives (Ewles and Simnett, 1995). Prochaska and DiClemente's (1982) model of transtheoretical changes has offered a means of understanding processes through which individuals' health behaviour may develop alongside changes in their own self-concepts. Importantly, such a model may be used by women to reflect on their perceptions of changes in their own health actions and to review the consequences and choices open to them in terms of their own identities. The importance to individuals of their own beliefs about health and their self-efficacy in guiding their behaviour is underlined by the influential extended Health Beliefs model advanced by Rosenstock et al. (1988). However, approaches which mainly focus on the individual have been criticized for not taking sufficient account of how the empowerment of individuals is intimately linked to power structures within communities and the wider society. The work of medical sociologists such as Blaxter (1990) in examining the relative influence of lifestyle changes, as compared with socio-economic structural factors such as housing and income, points up how little scope there may be for lifestyle changes, and how little relevance such changes may have for individuals' perceptions of their health chances if they cannot overcome fundamental social and material disadvantages. The work of Tones (Tones and Tilford, 2001) in developing a model for the analysis of health action, endorses the need for a multi-level perspective which views health action as an interactive outcome of individual experiences and perceptions, relationships and resources within communities and engagement in the development of wider social policies. The relevance of such approaches to the kinds of issues in understanding women's health raised in this chapter is clear. Their particular applicability is demonstrated in community-based health promotion projects such as that of Gibbons and Cazottes' groups in Nepal with both literate and non-literate women's groups (Gibbons and Cazottes, 2001). However, taking account of interdisciplinary perspectives can further enrich such understandings and dialogues if undertaken in a reflexive and dynamic way.

Insights from the management of specific types of complex risks may be useful for promoting such dialogue. We suggest the following, adapted from Buckley's work in managing violence (Buckley, 1999: pp. 102–3). Such a framework would encompass the following processes at an individual or group level:

- examining the nature of specific risks and reasons for taking them;
- exploring the whole context for potential outcomes in terms of who might benefit or be harmed by them;
- assessing what resources are available for controlling or managing risks;
- ascribing empowered rather than victim roles to women;

- encouraging the development of a sense of self which is resistant to stereotypic labels;
- facilitating processes of dialogue and feedback in which an overview can be taken;
- identifying and facilitating peer networks to promote mutual support and work towards change.

The range of insights for building women's health, presented by the contributors to this book, reflects a number of shared themes. They also point to the wealth of connections to be made with diverse groups of women, whose health problems and contributions to health may be variably visible in different societies, institutions and settings. A framework which assumes multiple viewpoints and interdisciplinary resources, can be used to facilitate constructive dialogues about health risk management, with and between women, so as to respect their management of their everyday lives.

Acknowledgements

We are most grateful to Anne Squire for her comments on the relevance of health models to this discussion.

Part I

'A Picture of Health': Women's Health in Historical Context

1
Images of Women's Health and Healing: Cultural Prescriptions?

Victoria Harris

We live in a culture in which it is still possible to ascertain categorical differences between the sexes, such that men can take professional, scientific roles in which they examine and in which women may become the object of examination through their sexuality and their relegation to relatively trivialized roles. Within such a culture, polarized images of women as healers and men as doctors have had a continuing historical existence which reflects and is embedded within a number of enduring themes in gender relations pertaining to health, medicine and caring. This chapter explores how such images may have been reinforced, so helping to provide a context for placing the kinds of health issues and actions raised in later chapters.

Gender here refers not to sex but to a cultural representation of a bipolar construction for obtaining and retaining meaning within natural existence: light/dark; Yin/Yang; life/death; Mars/Venus; hot/cold; male/female. Such polarities are given particular significance in terms of health where, from antiquity, it was believed that good health was to be achieved by finding an equilibrium involving opposing and complementary forces. Among the Hippocratics and others, 'The medical concept of balance, like the general notions of moderation, presupposed the existence of polarities and sets of extremes between which a mean must be sought' (Cadden, 1993: p. 17). Where there was imbalance, there was disorder. Where there was disorder, there was dis-ease of some description, with possible consequences beyond the individual: 'Something is rotten in the state of Denmark' (Shakespeare, *Hamlet* I.iv). So, acting both to maintain order and also, in sustaining culturally appropriate role divisions, to reinforce that order, has been embedded within the often gender-related health roles of doctors and healers.

'Doctor' in terms of our contemporary understanding of a public, professional health-related activity, dates back to only the nineteenth century. The immediate, non-professional responsibility for the health care of others has been, for much longer, differently organized and, along with personal care work in the domestic domain, within the provenance of women (Stacey, 1988). Indeed, it was not until the Flexner Report, published in 1910, that the basis of new medical accreditation standards, benchmarking a foundation in basic science, was established (Nesse and Williams, 1996). Nevertheless, to some extent, the older tradition of female health care can still be said to endure. In Western countries, the taking up and acting on alternative or complementary treatments which may be described as more concerned with 'healing' – as opposed to 'doctoring' as a kind of engineering applied to the body – have largely been undertaken by women. This tradition is a continuation of the role of healer for which we have early descriptions such as those set out in a twelfth-century handbook of gynaecology written by Dame Trotula of Salerno (LaBarge, 1986). Unfortunately, this guide to medicine for the use of women in this field has been lost, with male authors later taking up the occupation of her text.

Such appropriation of female knowledge by male 'scientific' practitioners is not unfamiliar. However, it has not entirely suppressed the enduring tradition of female healing knowledge. *The Principles of Chinese Medicine* is a relatively recent introduction and guide for the lay reader, prepared and written by a woman (Hicks, 1996). In it, numbers of citations by patients about treatment and of case studies of patients more often represent women (35) than men (14). The immediate impression is of substantially more women than men concerning themselves with health and medical practice not associated with the western scientific procedures developed over the last three centuries. This resonates with contemporary practices, where women rather than men have more frequently shown enthusiasm for exploring the efficacy of less invasive, herbal and therapeutically based treatments for ill-health. This is not to overlook men's increasing interest in alternative/complementary medical treatments. Nor is it to deny great differences in the type and severity of conditions to be treated. So, for instance, the treatment of a brain tumour is currently unlikely to be effective in the absence of the invasive techniques of neurosurgery and radiography.

An instruction manual written in the early 1390s by an elderly Parisian provides

> an interesting, if idealised, picture of a medieval *bourgeoise* busy about her daily tasks. These centred upon the care of her husband

with particular emphasis upon the need for cleanliness and proper food. But she is also supposed to assume responsibility for the health and well-being of their domestic staff. 'If one of your servants falls ill ... do you lay all common concerns aside, and do yourself take thought for him full lovingly and kindly ... seeking to bring about his cure'. A large section of the tract is devoted to gardening, partly because the lady of the house had to supply fruit and vegetables for the kitchen and see that their employees were adequately fed. Of equal importance, however, was the need to cultivate a fully stocked *herbier* so that all the necessary ingredients for routine medicaments and prophylactics lay immediately to hand. (Rawcliffe, 1995: p. 183)

Whatever may have been the case in the social and political spheres during the period of classical antiquity, in the sphere of reproduction in the Hippocratic medical tradition, the male/female polarity was not hierarchical. Here, both men and women were perceived as possessing 'seeds' of equal value, with the image of the female being that of collaborator and partner, of an equivalent significance to the male:

> In his treatise *On the Nature of the Child*, Hippocrates writes: 'If the sperm of both [parents] makes its way into the woman's womb ...' This model of reproduction ... suggested parallel functions of female and male and used the basic polarities of quality without denigrating the female partner ... it involves an abstract theory of balance and a set of concrete instructions, many but not all of which are clearly related to the notion of balance. It offers both a view of conception in which the sexes are on a par with each other and a massive amount of material based on the premise that female health is bound up with organs and functions that have no counterpoint in the male. (Cadden, 1993: p. 18)

Here, clearly, is some recognition of equivalence and difference, which is reiterated through historical accounts and contemporary experience. This responds to and reorganizes the perennial and elemental question of what constitutes and distinguishes 'the same' and 'the other', here male/female, for the purposes of sustaining a manageable order attainable at both individual and social levels. Thus, the creation of imagery to support (and if necessary impose) social and personal regulation becomes unavoidable. One may think of Louise Bourgeois's 'Spider' sculpture, on show during the opening year of the Tate Modern gallery. Given further force by natural history television programmes whose representations of the 'Black Widow' spider send shivers down the childhood spine, our response might be to view this as an icon of the terrifying female *fons et origo* of consuming oblivion, tying the hapless male to the bridal train of reproduction and death.

The view of women as the predominant healers has existed over millennia. This letter from the son of a famous herbalist, Margery Paston, illustrates the trust in female-prepared unguents and herbs to cure, rather than resorting to the surgeon's knife:

> He is the man that brought yow and me togedyrs, and I had lever then a xl li ye kond with your playster depart hym and hys peyne ... ye must send me wryghtyng hough it sold abyd on hys kne vnremevyd, and houghe longe the playster wyll laste good, and whethyr he must lape eny more clothys a-bowte the playster to kepe it warme or nought.

> [He is the man who introduced us, and I'd give more than £40 if you could take his pain away with your plaster ... you should write to me about how it has to stay on his knee, how long it will last, and whether or not he has to wrap any more cloths around the plaster to keep it warm]. (Cited in Rawcliffe, 1995: p. 185)

This idea of women holding the key to healing is further illustrated by tales of man divided both metaphorically and physically, representing good and evil in the personal and body-politic who can be made whole again only by women. Tales of such women include the old nurse Sebastiana, who is banished to a leper colony by a knight she had formerly cared for, now suffering both bodily and moral division. Her herbal skills enable her both to survive and, finally, to restore him to full health and well-being (Rawcliffe, 1995: p. 70).

None the less, the 'wise woman' as healer or prescient foreteller has often been pushed to the margins of society – often literally to the outskirts of towns and villages. From here it is an easy transition for those considered as 'other' to be transformed into witches or outcasts. Despite this, such outcast women were often consulted *in extremis* when children, relations or livestock were sick or needed specialist advice. The so-called 'back street abortionist', the local fortune teller, even the old woman living at the end of the street (whom local children might ridicule as a 'witch') are present-day relics of this tradition. Such women have taken huge personal risks in order to provide healing services to those in need.

Men, too, can be healers, but only very recently could women be doctors or even gynaecologists. Most hospital specialists, including gynaecologists, are men, reflecting women's difficulty in combining family life with demanding hospital careers. Healing and doctoring imply two quite different things, crucial to the history of the imagery and treatment of women and their participation in the development of modern medicine: healing is about a person; doctoring is about a patient:

> Women's experience of gynaecology was never regarded as important. Women were essentially and exclusively patients. (Dally, 1991: p. 124)

There is nothing necessarily malign about this distinction between healing and doctoring. However, in the former case, those in receipt of treatment are subjects, almost companions. In the latter, they are objects, relatively helpless, passive experiencers of both their own malady and its treatments. Moreover, what was insidious was the eighteenth- and nineteenth-century professionalization of doctoring as an exclusively male occupation.

Healing is something to be done *with* someone; doctoring is something to be done *to* someone. There is a powerful polarity which, again, is gendered. Neither set of relations needs be hierarchically placed, as better or worse, in relation to each other. Both have their more or less useful and useless procedures and purposes. They have their human meanings, and sometimes their inhuman ones, as with Macbeth's witches' linking certain ingredients to poison:

> Adder's fork, and blind-worm's sting,
> Lizard's leg and howlet's wing,
> For a charm of powerful trouble,
> Like a hell-broth, boil and bubble...

> (*Macbeth* IV.i)

or the experimental work conducted by Mengele and others at Auschwitz and elsewhere in Nazi-occupied Europe. Despite such extreme examples of unethical conduct, the skills and knowledge appropriate to medicine have to confront competence and incompetence, success and failure and the non-polarities of the unknown and unpredictable, the miraculous remission and the inexplicable demise.

Clarissa Estês, a Jungian analyst, refers to one of Woman's psychic tasks as:

> learning to make fine distinctions in judgement, sorting the mildewed corn from the good corn ... The mildewed corn has two meanings. As liquor, mildewed corn may be used as both an inebriative and a medication. There is a fungal condition called corn-smut – a rather fuzzy black fungus which is found in mildewed corn – which is also reputed to be hallucinogenic. (Estês, 1992: p. 99)

The notion of healing as collaboration and doctoring as mastery generates two radically different images and modes of relationship to the world and nature. One condition aspires to influence, the other to power. In Jordanova's analysis of the 1927 film *Metropolis* she points out that the fact that its scientist is male 'is essential not only to the plot but to the sexual dynamic that is integral to power over nature' (Jordanova, 1989: p. 125). She also cites other examples of this phenomenon, from Shelley's *Dr Frankenstein* to Hawthorne's Aylmer in *The Birthmark*. If women are perceived as the promontories of nature in the realm of social cultures dedicated to the 'mastery over nature' of scientific progress, then it follows that women, too, must be mastered. On this view, men are jealous and fearful of Woman's ultimate powers of generation. Frankenstein seeks to gain that power through his trained capacity as maker of an organism in God's image. The experiment goes horribly wrong; the 'monster', in his bewilderment, pulls the head from a child as if it were a daisy.

As such themes mesh, proving difficult to disentangle, they may often provide the energies for social transformation:

> We can learn something about the complexity, fragmentation, and difference of what we call 'sexuality' in the Middle Ages when we refrain from lending coherence to this multiplicity by our use of unifying terminology. (Cadden, 1993: p. 7)

The evolution of Natural Philosophy led to a kaleidoscopic range of disciplines routinely described as science, a term derived from the Latin *scientia* (knowledge). We might imagine this term to be neutral, except that history, including biomedical history, has recorded the writings and activities of men, and the language Latin was rarely learned by women. Their knowledge was recorded differently in the form of the vernacular, often in poems and songs which were easily memorable. Hence, women scarcely feature, except disproportionately in the records of medical/surgical developments in the eighteenth and nineteenth centuries as patients and 'guinea pigs' – not as practitioners or theorists commanding respect, even when they may have made outstanding contributions to medicine (Dally, 1991).

The capabilities usually and arguably associated with science – analytical thought, rationality, objectivity – have been claimed as attributes of Man, not of Woman, as a consequence of woman's perceived greater subjection to the despotism of biology. Menstruation, pregnancy, childbirth, menopause – experiences wholly unavailable to man, except as witnesses – liberated Man from such ineluctable and repeating 'natural' processes. They detached him, allowed a certain distance, the 'objectivity' that is a rhetorical prerequisite of the scientific project, although men are not entirely free of the exigencies of nature, being born and having to eat, excrete and die. This may be one of the factors contributing to the long and complex traditions of misogyny.

Woman, through the cycles associated with reproduction, repeats the ineradicably biological themes of life *in life* and so becomes a souvenir of death, a living *memento mori* at Man's side, intimately, domestically, in a host of virtually inescapable contexts. Men are shyer of a *memento mori*, which signifies that there can be no 'mastery' over Nature's strongest hand, namely Death. In some societies, women will wear nothing but black in public following the death of a loved one. Germaine Greer writes movingly of a Sicilian friend who, at the death of her mother, would

'Every day ... sit by the grave'. And who, as a further mark or genuflection in the face of mortality, 'put her bright-coloured scarves away and wore a black one'. (Greer, 1991: p. 316)

Of course, men have the capacity to grieve but without having to apply to themselves such a constant and systematic reminder through grief of their own mortality.

In contradistinction to women, who are cyclically subject to 'it/Her' and where gynaecological inspection is presumed to be an almost necessary commonplace, men may be more reticent and evasive about any institutional, and therefore public, confirmation of the bodily encroachments that may signify the end of living. Men's approximate equivalent of gynaecology, urology, is, all but a non-subject. Not for them the triennial letter summoning them to have yet another 'smear' test. Even the term 'smear' implies indignity: slugs and snails leave smear trails; prison cell walls can be 'smeared' in faecal matter. As for 'scrape', the very violence intrinsic in the term is enough to set one's teeth on edge.

Such reticence amongst the majority of males reveals otherwise hidden, unspoken and disagreeable vulnerabilities – the clothes in this case may come in white:

> Men also experience embarrassment and shame at the prospect of urological examination. It is a little embarrassing ... Not to the doctor it isn't. Whatever symptoms you have, you may be sure that the doctor will have seen it many times before. There really is nothing to be scared about: nevertheless, men are reluctant to admit to problems 'down there' for fear of modesty. (Apple, 1997: p. 54)

In considering the term 'Natural Philosophy', we can have no difficulty in imagining, and therefore considering, women to be key practitioners because of their role as healers: seeking herbs; identifying significant plants and animal tissue and appropriate locations for these to be found; accumulating wisdom in the use of medicinal preparations and their applications, observing, analysing. No doubt, illiteracy and political and educational underprivilege have contributed to this failure of historical acknowledgement and to the creation and sustaining of the myth of Woman's irrationality. However, it may well also have contributed to a loss of real knowledge through the absence of written records of what was used, how and for what maladies, as in the case of Dame Trotula. Thus, an important discipline in its own right and a large body of medically significant findings have been forgotten.

Public status would therefore be attributed more rarely to women healers. This echoes still in the scepticism of practitioners of conventional Western medicine about what survives or has been rediscovered of remedies derived from a rural and agrarian 'science', in which sound observation must have been crucial and 'peer review' spoken, immediate and made to be remembered down the generations of women born within a given community – a tradition still existing in many African societies (see, for instance, Vaz, 1997).

The development of biomedical science, with its Hellenic, rationalist substratum, eventually put paid to serious respect for this form of healing practice, allowing the medical profession, by the nineteenth century, to usurp women's traditional role in caring for the sick and supporting the idea that the 'normal' state of women was to be sick or diseased (Dally, 1991), providing a constituency of ready-made patients. William Blake expressed this concern in *The Sick Rose*:

> O Rose, thou art sick!
> The invisible worm
> That flies in the night,
> In the howling storm,
> Has found out thy bed
> Of crimson joy:
> And his dark secret love
> Does thy life destroy.

> (Blake, 1791–2: p. 213)

Women were also perceived as being incapable of the orderly practice of scientific medicine through 'their lack of analytical modes of thought' (Jordanova, 1989: p. 37).

The polarity represented by Woman, her ways and her knowledge, were thus rendered into the 'civilizing' shibboleth of the 'feminine'. In so far as she could not 'master' Nature, Woman could be transformed into a figure ironically with the emotional and moral function of civilizing the patriarchal social realm, acting upon the conscience of men to require their good behaviour rather than scientific, economic or political progress (Jordanova, 1989: p. 37).

This continues the notion of the healthy and 'inevitable' polarity obtaining to a social balance. Again, in her analysis of *Metropolis* Jordovana writes:

> The real business of life, whether it is labour or running Metropolis, is done by men, yet they lack some essential element to make them whole, and it is this ingredient which good feminin-ity can contribute. So that reason and sentiment can be seen as opposed to one another, they are also complementary (Jordanova, 1989: p. 130)

However, the context in which this moral arrangement is enacted and the structures arising from them are quintessentially industrial and therefore a condition of the eighteenth and nineteenth centuries and pre-world war twentieth century. None the less, the woman healer of the Middle Ages was not entirely lost to the male-dominated and largely male-sponsored scientific/medical developments (and establishments) around her:

> The country woman who practised herbal healing in addition to her agricultural and household duties was not likely to meet up with a professor of medicine from an urban university. (Cadden, 1993: p. 5)

But a certain complementarity, or what one might call an 'interdisciplinarity,' could take place:

> the herbalist might supply an apothecary in a nearby town who worked with practitioners who, though, they might not themselves know Latin, were anxious to acquire knowledge and prestige by attending a physician called in from the city to treat or advise a member of the local elite. (Cadden, 1993: p. 5)

However, moving from the medieval world-view closer to our own time, we find that with an increasing development and professionalization of biomedical practice, a male hegemony was once again established:

> The subject and practice of gynaecology ... developed during the second half of the 19th-century, the very period of maximum prejudice against women, when attitudes towards them were at their most bizarre, in a curious mixture of contempt and idealisation. (Dally, 1991: p. xvi)

The healing–doctoring polarity can still be seen in any hospital, where the most visible and predominant role of women in the treatment process is that of nurse, men being doctors or consultants. Such an imbalance has, in more recent times, begun shifting towards a greater parity.

Nevertheless, there remains the image, if not the unassailable fact, of a hierarchy largely composed of women in service-demarcated and utilitarian uniforms taking temperatures, changing beds, ensuring the proper consumption of medicines, turning the bodies in the bed, managing the means of disposal of bodily waste, checking, but not formally *examining* well-being. On the other hand, it is nearly always men (as consultants) who will appear as the occasional figures of definitive authority, whose uniform is a suit that can be worn on the street, on the train or at board meetings. The reality is not so cut-and-dried – we use the imagery of nurse and consultant as living archaeological fragments by which we construe a kind of society and its manifestations:

> One of the most marked features of the organisation of doctors into a profession was the exclusion of women and the insistence that they participate only in subservient tasks. (Dally, 1991)

> All doctors were male until the beginning of this century, and though fifty per cent of students in medical schools up and down the country are now female, the majority of them will never end up as consultants in hospitals (a mere thirteen per cent of all consultants in the UK are female) ... (Neuberger and Kyle, 1991: p. 164)

This is not to deny that hospitals, GPs' surgeries and the rest of the universe of professional Western medical intervention, also display to the laity a bewildering array of hierarchies, uniforms and functions. Furthermore, they are all in a state of flux, technologically and socially, through both internal and external forces and continually evolving economies and policies.

Nevertheless, the archaic and unchanging still persist in the imagination. Hearing the word 'nurse', most people may well form the image of Woman, and hearing the word 'doctor', the image of a man is formed. Jordanova, already cited here, supports this key point:

> Science and medicine have acted as mediators of ideas of nature, culture and gender, with verbal and visual images as the tools of that mediation. One of the most powerful aspects of scientific and medical constructions of sexuality is the way in which apparently universal categories were set up. These implied that there were profound similarities among all women to a much lesser extent than among men. (Jordanova, 1989: p. 42)

A familiar game in lateral thinking can still catch out people who have not heard it before. A father and son are in a motor accident. The father is killed and the boy is rushed to hospital for surgery. The surgeon on entering the operating theatre announces 'That's my son'. The most convoluted explanations are offered by listeners to solve this apparent conundrum, bringing on a veritable parade of vicars, milkmen and illegitimate siblings. The fact that such a simple, clear fable with a preposterously obvious explanation – that the surgeon is his mother – *exists* and still has the capacity to *bewilder* men and women alike, remains a vivid testimony to the power of the imagery that accrues around the placing of man and woman in the domain of health care.

The emergence of a middle class in a newly industrialized society saw the middle-class woman developing into a professional housewife. From this development came the image of the professional housewife. This often 'pale and frail' figure is described by Susan Sontag:

> TB was one index of being genteel, delicate, sensitive. With the new mobility (social and geographical) made possible in the eighteenth century, worth and station are not given; they must be asserted. They were asserted through new notions about clothes (fashion) and new attitudes toward illness. Both clothes (the outer garment of the body) and illness (a kind of interior decor of the body) became tropes for new attitudes toward the self. (Sontag, 1978: 78)

The new role manipulation of women was simply a step on the same journey towards excluding women from the public domain, to make them other, victims trapped in their own houses. Part of this entrapment was through weakness and illness. Women were debilitated, isolated, infantilized, as noted 200 years ago in Wollstonecraft's powerful critique of the social position of women:

> Men, indeed, appear to act in a very un-philosophical manner when they try to secure the good conduct of women by attempting to keep them always in a state of childhood. (Wollstonecraft, cited in Shearer, 1987: p. 914)

More diffuse and, it might be argued, more fluid and complex views of the male/female polarity seem to have prevailed in the Middle Ages, in relation to health care, where illiterate, rural Woman and literate, urban Man shared a mediated complementarity:

> the vast and evolving body of knowledge which constituted medieval medicine and natural philosophy ... did not offer a single model of the sexes, much less one which could be said to shape or to be derived from a clear system of gender roles. (Cadden, 1993: p. 2)

This remained true, to a certain extent, in the biomedical domain until relatively recently. During the seventeenth and eighteenth centuries:

'the subject of women's diseases was not a separate speciality. It was part of general surgery or else dealt with by a physician'. (Dally, 1991: p. 7)

In many agricultural societies, such as in Latin America, the past is often still close to the present. Over the centuries, different cultural traditions of healing have existed side-by-side with Christianity; the occult, modern medicine and spiritual healing interwoven into a 'multidisciplinary' whole. This continues in 'developed' countries, with an increasing acceptance of alternative beliefs, medicines and therapies:

The question: Cherie Blair is said to see Ayurveda specialist Bharti Vyas and Madonna has daily yoga sessions. So what can such complementary therapies offer pregnant women?

(Joanna Moorhead describing complementary therapies, in *The Guardian*, 10 May 2000, p. 10)

Werner (1995) suggests that the typical hierarchical pyramid system where the doctor is 'on top', should be developed into a lateral pyramid where the doctor is 'on tap' and 'the people come first'. This links well with the place of the traditional woman healer and the twenty-first century striving for a holistic form of medicine where the patient is much more part of the whole process.

In *The Rise of the Modern Urban Shaman* (2000), Staunton makes the point that:

Shamanism is non-hierarchical. There are no gurus to follow (or should not be) and no spiritual doctrine as such. A shaman does not worship nature; she honours, respects and feels part of the natural world. As I.M. Lewis has written: 'the entire shamanic community seems to assume that humans can participate in the authority of the gods'. (Staunton, 2000: p. 26)

Just as astronomers often practised astrology as part of their craft, so herbalists and physicians called on occult powers to assist them with their work. In a society in which religion, the occult, science, medicine and witchcraft were interchangeable, it was, for example, quite acceptable for religious leaders to 'prove' witches by the ducking stool. If they lived, they had used their occult powers to bring the forces of darkness to their aid. However, if they died, it 'proved' that they were innocent and vindicated by being drawn up to the heavenly kingdom.

Indeed, heavenly portents of one kind or another – thunder, lightning, comets, meteors – were the staple diet of pre-eighteenth-century Europe as well as other cultures. Along with 'alternative' medicine, such beliefs have returned to the present age alongside belief in 'ancient wisdom' or witchcraft, which has always been seen as persisting on the fringes of society.

Recently, political debate across Europe about the 'problem' of the Roma (or Romany) exemplifies how such inherited prejudices – and ambivalences – continue to be invoked. Roma people are often both consulted and rejected by the *gadje* (non-Roma). They are often viewed as pariahs and subjected to forced migration – usually at the instigation of local politicians assisted by the local press. They are sometimes viewed simply as purveyors of charms, amulets and talismans. However, in rural areas, Romany 'horse doctors' are still consulted for their ability to cure livestock, using secret knowledge, after orthodox veterinary treatment has failed. Roma women also believe in their power to heal and are still consulted – usually in secret in everyday life, but more openly at fairgrounds – to perform a healing ritual, tell a 'fortune' or put a curse (*amria*) on an enemy or rival. Fortune telling or casting spells, when practised by Roma women, is often seen as fraudulent by the authorities, who usually move them on. Forced migration – to the end of the street, out of the village, the town or the country or indeed, to ghettoisation in a special enclosure on the 'outskirts' – a site, a camp or 'reception centre' – has been a persistent solution for dealing with these aspects of 'the other', not least in the twentieth century and, so far, in the twenty-first. Romany identity is especially linked with problems seen as originating with 'new other' migrating peoples from Eastern European countries.

Tragically, from the same tradition and culture of both wisdom yet also of alienation and exploitation, more than 1,000 women are brought into Britain each year from Eastern Europe to work in sexual slavery.

> Women from the Balkan states … are charged thousands of pounds by criminal middle men for visas … often on the promise that they can pay off the balance of the fee in arrears by working for a few months in the sex industry or the 'entertainment business'. (Gillan and Ward, *The Guardian*, 30 May 2000, p. 4)

Despite the increasing number of women engaged in positions of power, including in medicine, there are still wide divergences between the images, roles and expectations of women as healers. Women seen as healers can still find themselves in positions of slavery and on the extremes of social existence.

Addressing such cultural ambivalence towards healing and its consequences is a task which raises challenges for the other disciplines discussed in this book: the therapeutic dialogues represented by counselling and psychotherapy; the empowerment and disempowerment made possible through the professions of medicine, law and nursing; the analytical perspectives provided by economics, sociology and statistics. The sanctioning of such women and the risk of damage to their own health, whether as witches, herbalists, healers, mothers or spiders, continues through apparently different but culturally equivalent symbolic forms. This chapter has aimed to set the historical scene for contemporary perspectives to continue the search for balance and resolution.

Acknowledgements

Dr Richard Davies and Peter Brinded are gratefully acknowledged for their assistance in researching this chapter.

Further reading

Dally, A., *Women under the Knife: A History of Surgery* (London: Hutchinson Press, 1991)

Jordanova, L., *Sexual Visions: Images of Gender in Science and Medicine between the 18th and 19th Centuries* (Madison: University of Wisconsin Press, 1989)

Rawcliffe, C., *Medicine and Society in Later Medieval England* (Stroud: Sutton Publishing, 1995)

Shearer, A., *Woman: Her Changing Image: A Kaleidoscope of Five Decades* (Wellingborough: Thorsons, 1987)

2
Disordered Minds: Women, Men and Unreason in Thought, Emotion and Behaviour

Joan Busfield

Introduction

Psychiatric disorder – to use a broad term – has never, contrary to some suggestions (Showalter, 1987), been a distinctively female malady (Busfield, 1994), and it has been widely recognized that men, no less than women, can be diseased in mind as well as in body. None the less, there have always been important differences between male and female psychiatric disorder. First, there have been differences between men and women in the typical patterns of disorder, generating a gendered landscape of psychiatric disorder changing over time (Busfield 1996, pp. 13–30). This gendering can be seen quite clearly in Table 2.1, which sets out data from a British survey of psychiatric disorder in the community.

Table 2.1 shows that, whereas the rates for functional psychoses – disorders of thought (of which schizophrenia is the most important) – are about the same for men and women, many other disorders show a marked gender imbalance. For example, phobias, anxiety and depression – disorders relating to emotional states – are more common in women than men. This is also the case for anorexia nervosa, at present the paradigmatic female mental disorder, not separately identified in this particular study. In contrast, many of the behavioural and personality disorders such as alcohol and drug-related disorders, as well as antisocial or dissocial personality disorder (again not specifically listed in this study), are more common in men. The findings of this study have been repeated in many others, and some studies additionally show how the pattern of symptomatology for a given condition also vary between men and women (see, for instance, J.M. Goldstein, 1992).

Table 2.1   Prevalence of psychiatric disorders by gender, adults 16–64

Rates per 1,000 in past week	Female	Male	Ratio F/M
Mixed anxiety and depression	99	54	1.8
Generalized anxiety disorder	34	28	1.2
Depressive episode	25	17	1.5
All phobias	14	7	2.0
Obsessive-compulsive disorder	15	9	1.7
Panic disorder	9	8	1.1
All neurotic disorder	195	123	1.6
Rates per 1,000 in past year			
Functional psychoses	4	4	0.0
Alcohol dependence	21	75	0.3
Drug dependence	15	29	0.5

NB: The two sets of rates cannot be added since, in one case, we have rates for the previous week and, in the other, rates per year.
Source: Meltzer et al. (1995).

Second, different causal accounts of psychiatric disorder are quite frequently offered for men and women. It was common in the nineteenth century to identify women's reproductive systems as having a major responsibility for any psychological disturbance they experienced. Women were generally held to be inferior to men and at the mercy of their biology, with menstruation, childbearing and menopause all assumed to make them potentially more mentally vulnerable and emotional, and more prone to psychological disturbance (Smith-Rosenberg, 1974). In contrast, though explanations of male disorder sometimes related to male biology, the understanding was very different. Men were seen less as the victims of their biology than as agents who could control their bodies through the exercise of will-power (Oppenheim, 1990; Shuttleworth, 1990).

In the twentieth century, such extremes of sexism were abandoned, but some of the old ideas remain, albeit in attenuated form. For example, for several decades until the 1960s, the condition of involutional melancholia was included in psychiatric classifications referring to a disorder of later life, particularly associated with women during the menopause (Jackson 1987: 207–11). Even more importantly, the more recent development of the disorder of premenstrual tension, and its incorporation into psychiatric classifications, shows the continuing importance of ideas about the impact of women's biology on their mental health, even thought they are no longer described in such obviously sexist terms.

Third, and related to this, there are differences in the typical treatments provided for men and women. For instance, women are given electro-convulsive therapy (ECT) more often than men (Donnelly, 2000) and are also more frequently prescribed psychotropic medication. In part this is because they are more often identified as having disorders for which these treatments are indicated, such as psychotic depression (for which ECT may be recommended) or anxiety and depression, where psychotropic drugs are widely prescribed. However, studies indicate that, even controlling for diagnosed condition, psychotropic drugs are more likely to be prescribed to women than to men (Ettore and Riska, 1993).

In this chapter, drawing on a range of sociological perspectives, I briefly explore the terrain of women and psychiatric disorder further, placing it in historical context and linking it to three domains: thought, emotion and behaviour (see also Busfield, 2002). I begin by examining key sociological perspectives in the field.

Sociological perspectives

Sociological scholarship on psychiatric disorder has been both extensive and diverse. I want briefly to consider five different perspectives.

Sociology of deviance

Perhaps the most influential and distinctively sociological approach to the terrain of psychiatric disorder has been to seek to understand it in terms of deviance and rule-breaking. Here, the focus is on the behaviours that lead an individual to be viewed as disturbed more than on the mental processes themselves. The approach can be traced back to Durkheim's (1964 [1895]) classic ideas about the normal and the pathological. Developing a functionalist perspective, Durkheim asserted society's fundamental need for rules – varying between societies and social groups – as a precondition of social order, and the consequent forces of social control involved in identifying individuals as deviant. This latter emphasis is particularly clearly represented in the work of labelling theories of deviance especially influential in the 1950s and 1960s, most notably in the case of psychiatric disorder in the work of Thomas Scheff (1999 [1967]). The deviance perspective, through its emphasis on the way concepts of mental health and illness change and vary over time, has come to be particularly associated with relativist claims about the categories and concepts of mental disorder. These emphasize their social construction – a loose phrase which is intended to highlight that categories, concepts and understandings are socially shaped.

Social epidemiology

Although an epidemiological approach to psychiatric disorder is not distinctively sociological, sociologists have made a major contribution to the analysis of the distribution of psychiatric disorders across populations. Notable here is the early study *Mental Disorders in Urban Areas* on the distribution of mental disorder in Chicago by sociologists Faris and Dunham (1965 [1939]), and the research of Hollingshead, a sociologist, and Redlich (1958), a psychiatrist, on the relationship between social class and mental disorder. This type of epidemiological work is intended to provide a foundation for research on the causes of mental disorder and has generated important explanatory studies such as Brown and Harris's study *Social Origins of Depression* (1978). While earlier sociological work tended to focus on the links between social class and psychiatric disorders, subsequent work has focused on gender, often under the influence of feminist ideas (for example, Gove, 1972; Smith, 1975), and on ethnicity (for example, Nazroo, 1997a).

Professionalization

Sociological work on professionalization, particularly grounded in Weberian ideas, has provided a very influential perspective on thinking about psychiatric disorders. Here the focus shifts to those given formal responsibility for dealing with these disorders – psychiatrists and other mental health professionals. The importance of such work lies not only in analysing the emerging power of psychiatric professionals, but also in understanding the way in which their activities, and practices shape mental health services as well as concepts of disorder, aetiological accounts and treatments. While much of the work in this tradition has focused on medicine in general, some has focused specifically on the terrain of psychiatry. Notable here is Scull's (1975) early work on asylum doctors, as well as the work of some social historians influenced by sociological ideas, such as Goldstein's (1987) study of the French psychiatric profession in the nineteenth century.

Political economy

Ideas derived from political economy, particularly Marxist ideas, have had a major impact on some sociological work on psychiatric disorder. On the one hand, they have helped to shape ideas about changing levels of psychiatric disorder over time, as for instance, in Navarro's

(1976) linking of capitalism and levels of health and illness, including mental and psychological problems, or Brenner's (1978) thesis that mental health is associated with the strength of the economy. These ideas have been further developed in Warner's (1994) work linking levels of mental illness to labour market needs. On the other hand, it has contributed to the analysis of both the development of the asylum and the move to community care, not only in Scull's (1977; 1979) well-known work, but also in more recent theorizing such as Goodwin's (1997), which draws on ideas about welfare regimes (Esping-Andersen, 1990).

Post-structuralism

The final sociological approach draws on the work of Foucault, especially his early text *Madness and Civilisation* (1967) and his later work on governmentality (1991a). Foucault and his followers have emphasized the inseparable link between power and knowledge and how power can have a productive and constitutive as well as repressive role (Miller, 1987). They have also emphasized the diffusion of psychiatric and psychological ideas and professionals across a range of sites beyond the asylum, forming what is described as a 'psy complex'. These ideas have influenced a number of social historians such as Lunbeck (1994). Post-structuralism is also associated with work on the sociology of the body (Turner, 1996) and the sociology of the emotions (Bendelow and Williams, 1998), both of which are beginning to be applied to the sphere of psychiatric disorder as well as being used in more mainstream sociology. For instance, Giddens (1991) discusses anorexia nervosa as an archetypal illness of late modern society.

I now deploy elements from these different perspectives to explore psychiatric disorder in women. My starting point, derived from Foucault (1967), is that the wide terrain of psychiatric disorder is best viewed as different forms of 'unreason' (see Busfield, 1996, pp. 69–75) which I distinguish here in terms of thought, emotion and behaviour.

Unreason in thought and behaviour in the nineteenth century

Nineteenth-century notions of insanity and lunacy were grounded, as in earlier centuries, in lay ideas about disturbed, irrational behaviour. The mad person was someone whose behaviour seemed not only unacceptable but also, in some way, irrational and inexplicable and whose thought was judged to be disturbed. Irrational behaviour stemmed from, and reflected, irrational thought.

Those identified as lunatics had long been regarded a problem, and had been dealt with in a variety of ways: some were to be found in private madhouses, workhouses or, from the second half of the eighteenth century, in voluntary asylums; some were held by their families, sometimes confined and even put in chains; others, especially if relatively harmless, became vagrants and beggars. The major development in the nineteenth century was the establishment of a system of publicly funded asylums for lunatics. These had a dual foundation. First, they were intended to serve as places of custody for persons whose irrational thought and behaviour was threatening to the social order, perhaps because they were violent, or because they were difficult or disruptive. Second, they were intended to be places of security (asylum in the sense of protection) and recovery for the individual. While the latter motivations were crucial in securing the necessary support for the initial establishment of asylums, as the century progressed, the custodial role of the asylums became increasingly predominant and they became large-scale, regimented institutions offering little in the way of therapy.

Voluntary and public asylums were the locations where the new speciality of medicine, psychiatry, developed as asylum doctors began to form associations to discuss and further their common interests, and set up journals to share their ideas. Throughout much of the century, the categories of mental disease with which these new specialists operated were those inherited from previous centuries – chiefly mania, melancholia and dementia, with others, such as hysteria and epilepsy, also used. However, by the end of the century, classification was seen as one way the asylum doctors could assert their new professional identity and, as a result, new categories began to be introduced. Kraepelin's (1896) ground-breaking distinction between two types of psychosis – manic-depressive psychosis and dementia praecox (soon to be renamed schizophrenia) – was first introduced in the final decade of the century, and the language of psychosis became the language in which notions of lunacy and madness were delineated by psychiatrists in the twentieth century.

Given the focus on controlling irrational, sometimes dangerous behaviour, it is not surprising to find that as many men as women were confined in the new asylums, but their treatment, using the term in its broadest sense, was not identical. Women, for instance, were more likely than men to be described as having melancholia and the category of hysteria (initially understood as a condition resulting from movement of the womb) was almost exclusively applied to women, many medical men believing that it only occurred in women. In contrast, men were far more likely than women to be detained within the asylum on the grounds that their criminal behaviour was the product of lunacy, and the dominant image of the criminal lunatic was male (Busfield, 1994). Indeed, when special institutions for criminal lunatics began to be set up in the second half of the nineteenth century (Broadmoor was the first in Britain in 1863), they confined mostly men. The only significant female image of the criminal lunatic was of women who committed infanticide (Smith, 1981).

Another very significant gender difference came in the explanatory accounts that were offered for women's mental disturbances. For instance, women who killed their children were often seen as doing so because of the physiological changes associated with childbirth. Similarly, accounts of melancholia stressed the role of the ovaries on women's minds and behaviour. Furthermore, there was strict separation of men and women within the asylum, and the work assigned those considered fit enough followed the prevailing gender division of labour, with male inmates assigned work in the gardens and on the estate, whereas female inmates contributed to the domestic work of the asylums, including working in the laundries.

Unreason in emotion in the twentieth century

Throughout the nineteenth century, doctors dealt with mental health problems outside the asylum as well as within it. However, in the second half of the nineteenth century, when psychiatry began to develop on the foundation of asylum practice as a more distinctive speciality of medicine, some doctors were also increasingly beginning to specialize in treating less severe psychological problems outside the asylum, the two areas of work intersecting and feeding on one another. This 'office psychiatry' as it has been termed, was founded on rather different principles from asylum psychiatry. In asylums, the custodial dimension of practice was strong: individuals in asylums were legally detained, often against their wishes, frequently at the behest of others, including the police and courts. In contrast, individuals seeing doctors privately at their own home, or in the consulting room, typically had less severe psychological problems and received treatment on a legally voluntary basis, often referring themselves, or being encouraged to seek help by a family or friend. Consequently therapeutic motivations were more dominant and self-referral was more important.

It is in this sphere of office psychiatry that we find a growing concentration of specialists on the realm of the emotions and on irrationalities of emotion – fears, anxiety, misery – rather than on irrationalities of thought and behaviour. Individuals with such problems were not 'mad' in either the lay or medical sense – their thought and behaviour seemed generally rational – yet their feelings and emotions were disturbed and somehow 'unreasonable' – out of proportion, not fully within their control, and apparently beyond the powers of reason. That such problems should be brought to medical attention was not new, for doctors had long tried to treat the 'troubled in mind' (MacDonald, 1981). What was new was the development of specialist practice around this area of work. Moreover, at the end of the nineteenth century and the beginning of the twentieth century, the new specialists were at least as active as their asylum counterparts in developing new categories of disorder. For example, neurasthenia, or 'nervous exhaustion', was introduced by Beard in America in 1869 to describe a diffuse range of symptoms, many of which had a clear bodily component, such as insomnia, flushing and drowsiness. But Beard (1972 [1881]) emphasized other symptoms that were more obviously psychological and related to the emotions, such as a range of fears: for example, fear of open and closed spaces, fear of being alone and fear of responsibility. Even more influential was the work of Freud (see, for instance, Freud, 1977 [1905]), who introduced the concept of psycho-neurosis (which he contrasted with actual neurosis) to cover a range of conditions of psychogenic origin, such as anxiety neurosis and obsessional neurosis. Most of the psycho-neuroses were delineated in terms of pathologies of feeling and emotion, and were assumed to have emotional causes, originating particularly in unconscious mental conflict. But even when the symptoms were more behavioural, Freud emphasized the importance of feelings and emotions, often unconscious, in their causation, as in the case of hysteria. The inner world of feelings was brought centre stage.

Whereas Freud focused on disorders such as hysteria, anxiety neurosis, phobias and obsessions, other writers, such as Adolf Meyer in America, paid more attention to depression (Jackson, 1987, pp. 195–8), and a contrast began increasingly to be made between the more severe, psychotic (or endogenous) depression and the less severe, neurotic (reactive) types of depression – the latter term being first used in an American psychiatric classification in 1935 (Jackson, 1987: p. 117).

This growing interest in different forms of depression underpinned the increasing use of terms such as 'mood disorders' or 'affective disorders'. The concept of affective disorders still features in both the American Psychiatric Association's *Diagnostic and Statistical Manual*, now in its fourth edition (DSM-IV) (1994), and *The ICD-10 Classification of Mental and Behavioural Disorders* (World Health Organisation, 1992). However, as it did when first introduced, it refers specifically to types of depression and does not include other disorders defined in relation to emotions such as anxiety states and phobias.

It was within this new terrain of the emotion-related disorders – the psycho-neuroses including reactive depression – that women increasingly became the object of specialist psychiatric attention. In several cases, the initial formulations centred on men rather than women. For instance, neurasthenia, seen by Beard (1972 [1881]) as a disease of civilization, was initially constructed around men and was linked to a lack of nerve-force in some of them. However, since women, through the construction of femininity, tended to be seen as, almost by definition, lacking in will-power, it was women rather than men who came to be increasingly regarded as neurasthenic. The psychiatric disorder of shell-shock which was delineated in the First World War, and later reformulated and amplified into the broader category of war neuroses, was also a male mental disorder. Although, for obvious reasons, it was usually applied to men, it helped to gain acceptance for psychological explanations of psychiatric disorder.

However, the new understandings of the impact of inner mental conflict were subsequently applied more frequently to women than to men since generally women were held to be more psychologically vulnerable than men. They were also more willing to bring more problems centring on feelings to medical attention – feelings of anxiety, fear and loss – because to do so was not threatening to their identity as women. In contrast, admitting to psychological problems was threatening to conceptions of masculinity (Oppenheim, 1991). Consequently, the new concepts and explanatory ideas were readily applied to women who became, in practice, the major focus of specialist expertise outside the asylum, a specialist expertise becoming more diverse and now beginning to include the work of non-medical psychotherapists and psychologists. It was women more than men who were likely to receive the psycho-dynamic forms of therapy and to be diagnosed as having an anxiety neurosis. And further, with the revolution in psycho-pharmacology after the Second World War, it was women more than men who were more likely to be the recipients of the new tranquillizers in the 1960s and 1970s, and subsequent generations of drugs for depression such as Prozac. This put them at greater risk than men of becoming dependent on prescribed drugs. To some extent, the new drugs shifted attention away from mind and back to the body, yet, in terms of symptoms, the focus was still on emotions, even though psychiatric classifications began to eschew the concept of neurosis on the grounds of its aetiological assumptions. The new drugs also increasingly took the treatment of anxiety and depression (terms that are used almost interchangeably) away from the specialist, giving them instead to the general practitioner, who could prescribe the new drugs far more cheaply and quickly than the specialist. This seemed appropriate, since anxiety and depression had become the common mental disorders, whose incidence was far higher than that of psychotic disorders such as schizophrenia (Goldberg and Huxley, 1992).

Unreason and behaviour in the second half of the twentieth century

The earlier expansion of psychiatric work into the sphere of the emotions continued and flourished in the second half of the twentieth century and through into the twenty-first. Alongside this transformation came a further area of expansion of psychiatry into the so-called personality and behaviour disorders. We have already seen how the criminal lunatic was a key figure in public images of insanity in the nineteenth century, and various concepts were developed to encompass such figures. One was the notion of moral insanity, first used in 1835, to describe a disorder of both emotion and the will. Moral insanity was the precursor of the notion of psychopathic disorder – a term applied to individuals who persistently engaged in criminal acts and wrongdoing and seemed without guilt or conscience (Ramon, 1987). Further transformations led to the present-day concepts of antisocial personality disorder, delineated in the DSM-IV (American Psychiatric Association, 1994) and dissocial personality disorder, set out in the ICD-10 (World Health Organisation, 1992) as well as borderline personality disorder and conduct disorder (Manning, 2000). In parallel with these disorders, a range of other personality disorders were introduced, such as narcissistic, dependent and paranoid personality disorders, as well as sexual disorders and substance use disorders (drug and alcohol disorders), all often located under the now broad umbrella of personality and behaviour disorders.

What has largely disappeared in this process of transformation and amplification has been the linkage with irrational thought that was such an important feature of nineteenth-century notions of criminal insanity. Such notions are far less visible in the terrain of personality and behaviour disorders precisely because the range of these disorders has so expanded. Indeed, it has frequently been argued that these disorders do not belong to the category of mental disorders at all (Wootton, 1959) and, significantly, the DSM-IV now places personality disorders on a separate axis of its classificatory schema. The new personality and behaviour disorders have been framed less around irrational behaviour grounded in irrational thought than around behaviour held to be irresponsible or unreasonable and linked to longer-term behavioural and personality tendencies. The unreason at issue lies more in behaviour than in the thought that underlies it and the judgement is not one of 'madness' but of the unacceptability of behavioural and personality features. Significantly, too, there is relatively little attention to emotions within this domain, even though feelings such as anger may be involved in the violence that is a common feature of several of these disorders.

In contrast to the psycho-neuroses, personality and behaviour disorders tend to be a male rather than female territory, though there are some notable exceptions such as anorexia nervosa. Epidemiological studies typically show rates of drug and alcohol dependence twice as high in men as in women (see Table 2.1 above) and sexual and personality disorders are also more common in men. However, anorexia nervosa (listed as a developmental disorder in the DSM-IV but grouped as a behavioural syndrome associated with physiological disturbances and physical factors in the ICD–10), is, according to the DSM, nine times as common in women as in men.

Conclusion

This chapter has shown that the territory of psychiatric disorder has been and remains, a changing, shifting one. When psychiatry developed as a distinctive speciality in the nineteenth century, the focus was on irrational thought, and both men and women were to be found in the asylums. However, by the end of the century, specialist practice extended to the realm of feelings and emotions that were apparently not amenable to rational control, and more and more women were brought into its compass. However, the advent of psychotropic medication in the 1950s meant that treatment for the common mental disorders such as anxiety and depression became as much a task for the general practitioner as the specialist. In the second half of the twentieth century, specialist practice returned the focus to behaviour but moved away from an emphasis on irrational thought to the problematic, sometimes dangerous behaviour often associated with alcohol and drug problems, sexual problems, and personality disorders, which are much more a male territory. But it has not removed all attention from unreason in the realm of feelings and emotions. It is here, above all, where women have been viewed as distinctively disturbed and constructions of femininity and mental disorder have intersected.

It is difficult to predict the ways in which the current gendering of psychiatric conditions will change. The major changes occurring in the gender division of labour in paid employment are likely to have a significant impact on male and female behaviour and on expressions of distress. The focus of specialist mental health services is also likely to change over time. What is clear, however, is that the current focus on disturbed behaviour, and in particular on risk and danger to the public, is at present drawing increasing proportions of men into the mental health services. In so doing, it is rapidly undermining the female predominance that characterized much of the second half of the twentieth century. This change could have a number of benefits for women. On the one hand, it may lead to greater efforts to change male behaviour which may itself be the cause of much female distress, as when male violence within the family leads to anxiety and depression in women. On the other hand, it may also help to challenge assumptions that women are weaker and more vulnerable than men. Women have potentially as much to gain as to lose from recent developments in mental health practice.

Further reading

Busfield, J., *Men, Women and Madness: Understanding Gender and Mental Disorder* (London: Macmillan, 1996).

Ettore, E. and Riska, E., *Gendered Moods: Psychotropics and Society* (London: Routledge, 1993).

Prior, P., *Gender and Mental Health* (London: Macmillan, 1999).

Ussher, J., *Women's Madness: Misogyny or Mental Illness?* (London: Harvester Wheatsheaf, 1991).

Part II
Breaking and Building Bodies

3
Women and Deliberate Self-Harm
Rosie Doy

Introduction

The phenomenon of deliberate self-harm is relevant to women's health. This is because a significant number of women harm themselves and are not in contact with health services, and also because the behaviour is a symptom of their distress and disempowerment within their bodies and the wider psycho-social world. Its study provides a good illustration of the need to understand women's health and 'wellness' in its most holistic sense.

Estimates of population rates of self-injurious behaviour in Western countries vary between one in 150 and one in 100, of which 75–97 per cent relate to women's self-injury (Department of Health, 1992; Favazza, 1996; Jack, 1992; Tantam and Whittaker, 1992; Winschel and Stanley, 1991). Mental health nurses working in acute settings in the UK report that in their care groups it is mostly women who have issues around self-harm (Doy, 1995). Although men also deliberately self-harm, this chapter focuses on the majority experience of women.

Such ways of 'writing the body' to signal female distress have only recently become more visible, as they are usually undertaken secretly and shamefully. They have become more frequently recognized in the literature since the 1980s, but a perplexing array of terms and definitions obscures the distinction between the intentions of suicidal and deliberate self-harming behaviour and thereby the true extent of deliberate self-harming activities and associated distress in women's experience (Jack, 1992; Smith et al., 1998). The term suicide defines actions that lead to or are intended to lead to death (Hawton and Catalan, 1987). By contrast, deliberate self-harm means that a person hurts herself, either to signal distress or to release or manage overwhelming feelings (Burstow, 1992). At least three sets of 'voices' with competing discourses tell the stories of women and deliberate self-injury.

The first and historically most powerful discourse has emanated from medical and psychiatric professionals' theorizing and objectifying the behaviour and experiences of women. Self-harming behaviour has sometimes provoked frustration and annoyance in these professionals (Favazza and Conterio, 1988). This discourse treats self-harm as either 'attention-seeking', if the person is not deemed suicidal, or as an attribute of a personality disorder. Terms such as 'self-harm', 'self-injury', 'self-mutilation' and 'body abuse' are often used interchangeably by individuals using differing criteria. For example, a nurse may construe a cut on a patient's forearm as 'superficial scratching' and 'superficial self-harm', while her colleague may describe the same injury as a 'laceration' and discuss it in terms of 'self-mutilation' (Doy, 1995).

The second set of voices is that of the survivors, now louder as many have engaged in the political task of telling their stories, to be heard by health care professionals, of how damaging and abusive their 'care' may have been (Martinson, 1998; Pembroke, 1994).

A third set of voices is that of groups influenced by feminist research, theorizing and practice. It includes the 'survivors' movement, users of mental health services and groups. Such groups include the UK Bristol Crisis Centre, which is a charitable collective offering a range of services for women, with a strong focus on self-injury. This discourse emanates from women carers and professionals who are articulating new ways of understanding and working with women who choose to damage their bodies (Smith, 1998).

Reflecting these sets of voices, and some of the tensions between them, this chapter will first provide a brief overview of relevant literature. Second, it will present related themes emerging from the author's own research into self-harming women (Doy, 1995) which is particularly informed by psychoanalytic feminism, which emphasises the power and significance of interpersonal and intrapersonal processes surrounding deliberate self-harming. The conclusions consider some implications for sensitive, evidence-based service development.

Defining the problem

Different interest groups and discourses relate to deliberate self-harm by women. Clarke and Whittaker (1998) choose the emotive term 'self-mutilation' to describe deliberate self-cutting. While they argue that it is a 'succinct description', it is a term many women who self-cut find annoying (Martinson, 1998). Self-mutilation such as castration, attempts to amputate limbs and fingers, or gouging, are more characteristic of severe psychotic illness where injury results from deluded fixed beliefs or hallucinations concerning the person's body. This is different from self-harming. Therefore, this chapter will not refer to deliberate self-injuring behaviour as self-mutilation.

Another term sometimes linked with self-harm is 'self-poisoning', through ingesting substances, including legally obtained drugs. As this sometimes results in death it may be associated with suicide. However, the term 'suicide' is much contested in the self-harm context, as to whether the self-harming person intends or is motivated to die (Schneidman and Faberow, 1961). As a final act of deliberate self-harm, resulting in death, 'suicide' is more visible in official statistics. However, relying on rates of suicide as an indicator of self-harm may help render self-harming women invisible. The suicide rate of 4 per 100,000 women compared with 13 per 100,000 men in the UK population can only partly indicate the extent to which women self-harm. However, there is wide agreement in both the United Kingdom and Europe that women are twice as likely as men to be reported as either self-poisoning or self-injuring (Jack, 1992). To help clarify the reasons for this, the author carried out a qualitative interview study with mental health nurses with regular experience of women and self-injury (Doy, 1995).

Gender and self-harm

The notion that it is women who most often self-cut is reflected in the pattern of case examples offered in research (Burstow, 1992; Smith et al., 1998), published personal stories of self-harm (for example, Pembroke, 1994) and in the author's study of mental health nurses (Doy, 1995). However, Hawton and Catalan (1987) challenge the notion that women invariably predominate in self-cutting activity. In a report on admissions for 'deliberate self-injury' to a general hospital in Oxford between 1980 to 1984, nearly as many men (75 per cent) as women (86 per cent) were admitted with cuts to the wrist or forearm (Hawton and Catalan, 1987: 150–1).

Johnson and Britt (1967), reported high levels of self-mutilation in men's prisons including self-cutting and more bizarre and damaging injury. Tantam and Whittaker's (1992) behaviourally focused work on diagnosis of 'personality disorder' suggests that if men are separated from wider society and given a subsidiary position when sent to prison, they begin to show more 'feminine' cutting behaviours. It may be argued that disempowerment and subjection to incarceration in a patriarchal institution lead to an increase in self-cutting behaviours in both sexes. However, Garner and Butler (1994) argue that women are more likely than men to self-harm repeatedly while in-patients in secure health settings.

Since the mid-1990s, the literature on self-injury has focused increasingly on debates and evidence on treatment approaches provided by the standpoints of women themselves and of feminist-aware practitioners. It is set mainly within three theoretical frameworks: psychoanalytic, medical and feminist empathic.

Psychoanalytic theory

Psychoanalytic theorists trace the damaging behaviour of the adult to the early experiences of the baby and child. While Freud's theories have drawn criticism from many feminists for their biological essentialism, psychoanlytic feminism has found them liberating (Brennan, 1992; Mitchell, 1974; Tong, 1989) in attempting to explain women's oppression by analysing internal psychic processes. The mother/child relationship may be analytically related to women-identified attributes of warmth, empathy and relating to others, such that conflict and ambivalence in childhood may lead to self-harming behaviour in later stages of life (Tong, 1989). This standpoint thus raises a more empathic critical awareness of the dynamic processes in significant adult/child relationships and their links with interpersonal dynamics of vulnerability and defence within the relationship of therapeutic nurse-helper and patient.

Medical discourse

'Medical' or 'psychiatric' discourse has defined self-injury using a number of diagnoses over time, the most popular now being Borderline Personality Disorder (World Health Organization, 1994). Such a diagnosis is, arguably, a classificatory 'bin' for women's little-understood behaviours, leading to their being perceived as attention-seeking, hysterical or hard to manage (Smith et al., 1998). Such discourse tends to invalidate these women subjects by blaming them for their self-injuring symptoms and merely seeking to contain these difficult behaviours. The medical or psychiatric mode of understanding and treating deliberate self-injury seeks to re-educate and modify 'problem' behaviour (Pembroke, 1994; Smith et al., 1998) rather than to understand the deeper, personal and lived meanings generating self-injuring behaviours.

Women whose deliberate self-injuring has led to hospital admission have sometimes protested at their damaging treatment during such times of great personal distress (Pembroke, 1994). The medicalized, patriarchal stance taken by health care professionals in hospitals, rather than offering care and empathy, provides, for many women, an abusive and silencing experience.

Feminist empathic discourse

To understand both the position of women and the expression of their distress within current social institutions, many feminists argue for the need to apply a critical awareness of the patriarchal nature of gendered power relationships and hierarchies within society and within interpersonal encounters including medical and psychiatric relationships with women users of services. Many social constructions of femininity tend to diminish and label as negative, qualities such as caring, mothering, feeling and nursing (Smith, 1992). These are succouring attributes which are, paradoxically, undervalued in professional helping within health services currently dominated by doctors and psychiatrists.

My own experience as a former mental health nurse included working with women who self-injured deliberately and repetitively, often by self-cutting. In such work, I have personally experienced feelings of powerlessness and frustration springing from two sources. The first was a sense that belief in the importance of supporting such women was definitely against the grain of the psychiatric management and nursing team colleagues' manner of work with these women. The second emanated from a sense of ill-preparedness in my practice in the 1970s and 1980s, when deliberate self-injury by cutting was very poorly understood.

A feminist standpoint recognizes the interaction between social structures, the personal self, the dominant culture and use of language in the definition, diagnosis and treatment of a woman's distress (Abbott, 1990; Reinharz, 1992). These may shape distress in her early life, how her subsequent experience is interpreted and how far it is validated by others.

There is now wide agreement that body size, eating habits and disorders involving food are clearly linked to the position of women in society. Burstow (1992), among others, related the efforts of those who develop anorexia and bulimia nervosa to control their body size to the low self-esteem resulting from psycho-social processes which 'place' women and objectify women's bodies. Similar dynamics influence a woman who deliberately self-injures by cutting, where the only avenue apparently open to her to express her emotional experience is in using her body to make visible and bleeding marks. These serve to release feelings and communicate selfhood to others (Favazza, 1996; Pembroke, 1994; Smith et al., 1998).

Mental health nurses may be assumed to recognize self-injuring readily as both a symptom of past experience and as a coping strategy, given their professional value base emphasizing the therapeutic relationship, (w)holism and self-awareness in nursing relationships (Butterworth, 1994). However, the stories of women with experiences of self-injury frequently report quite the opposite reaction from mental health professionals involved in their care (Martinson, 1998; Smith et al., 1998).

The following quotation is from a book of survivor stories (Pembroke, 1994) written mainly by women who have lived with self-cutting and treatment within mainstream mental health services. These provided an early and powerful set of writings which countered the medical discourse:

> During my psychiatrisation ... [I tried] to achieve the elusive 'Appropriate Behaviour' but to no avail. I failed miserably at being a 'good patient'. Something was very wrong with the treatment but I didn't have the language or analysis to articulate it beyond refusing to co-operate with it ... It was treating distress as merely aberrant behaviour. (Pembroke, 1994: 32)

This quotation illustrates the dissonance created in one woman's experience between the prevailing medical reading of self-cutting and its power to prescribe the parameters of the behaviour expected of the 'good patient'. It reflects a theme within the collection that silencing and invalidation characterized the mental health services in the 1980s and the early 1990s.

In contrast, an 'empathic' discourse emphasizes relating, meanings, connections and growth as a two-way process between helper and woman. Psychoanalytic feminist and therapy perspectives and the stories of 'survivors' and service users can especially inform such a discourse. Empowering the woman, in supporting her to gain or maintain control and develop safer ways of coping with distress, is fundamental to this way of being with women who deliberately self-injure (Burstow, 1992). A nursing relationship informed by such a perspective emphasizes that the aim of interpersonal interactions is to support a client to gain her own insights into problems and treatments.

Unpacking deliberate self-injury

Words used to describe various types of deliberate self-harm include: deliberate self-mutilation, self- or body abuse, self-harm, attention-seeking and para-suicidal behaviour, with little agreement on their application to particular behaviours. Some involve aspects of physical injury as diverse as cultural marking and tattooing (Tantam and Whittaker, 1992); over-exercising (Burstow, 1992), self-mutilation arising from serious mental illness or other disorder, or self-injury arising from obsessional and ritualistic preoccupations (Favazza, 1989; 1996).

There remain great variations in ways of understanding, labelling and responding to such actions. For example, over-exercising and cultural tattooing may be viewed as positive or even fashionable, while self-cutting and mutilation may occasion horror or be intentionally ignored. Self-injury is culturally defined. Tattooing and other body adornment, entwined with rites of passage and cultural belonging, should be considered separately from deliberate-self injury as a signal of distress and dis-ease.

Some nurses and other helpers use the term 'body abuse' to refer to self-harming activities. However, this term conflates self-injurious activities including self-cutting, self-burning and problematic eating, even including other related categories of behaviour as abusive, including smoking and problem drinking.

In this chapter, concepts of deliberate self-injury or self-cutting which draw on a psychoanalytic feminist perspective are employed to describe self-harm where a woman uses marking and hurting parts of the body to cope with distressing feelings or to experience a sense of self.

What is deliberate self-injury?

Deliberate self-injury has been described as:

> the commission of deliberate harm to one's own body ... without the aid of another person, and the injury is severe enough for tissue damage (such as scarring) to result. Acts that are committed with conscious suicidal intent or are associated with sexual arousal are excluded. (Winschel and Stanley, 1991: 306)

Researchers have identified several common features including: a sudden impulse to harm oneself which feels impossible to resist; a build-up of feelings, for example frustration or self-loathing, which feels impossible to contain; a sense of lacking control; a reduction in the perception of alternatives: experienced coping ability and a surge of relief following self-injury (Kahan and Pattison, 1984; Miller, 1994).

The literature provides conceptual frameworks which often include terms and analysis of the degree of each self-injury as 'serious' or 'risky'. Descriptions of self-injury as 'serious' often include words that convey a sense that such activity encompasses some intention to die. Often, the taking of a non-fatal overdose, or the use of self-injury and cutting behaviour, is described as being less aggressive, less 'serious' than behaviour that is labelled as suicidal. However, *superficial or moderate* self-injury – described, for example, by Favazza (1996) working in American psychiatry – is the most common form of deliberate self-injury but is the least understood and is under-researched. This category can include cutting, burning, scratching, skin-picking, hair-pulling, hitting, picking at wounds. The most commonly reported form is cutting, most frequently, the wrists, upper arms and inner thighs. A tension in using such a framework is that, while providing a conceptual hierarchy of 'seriousness', it may also be used to rank the individual and her hurting.

Research into deliberate self-cutting

In the mid-1990s, I carried out a research study of experiences of nursing women who self-harm, particularly by cutting, at a time when community mental health services were limited. At that time there was a surge of deliberate self-harming behaviour seen in Accident and Emergency (especially self-poisoning by overdosing) and acute admission units, and health and social care literature highlighted self-cutting among young women as a problematic care issue (Clarke and Whittaker, 1998; Favazza, 1989; Hawton and Catalan, 1987).

The study involved semi-structured, individual, hour-long interviews with women mental health nurses, examples of the third set of voices described above. A random sample of ten registered mental nurses was selected from a hospital total of 35 female, qualified, day and night staff, on acute wards admitting women who deliberately cut. To ensure their voluntary participation and informed consent, each was provided with information, opportunity and time to discuss and consider the study's rationale and ethical framework. Care was thus taken not to place participants at a disadvantage by the researcher, aiming for a non-abusive feminist research approach (Reinharz, 1992). Each received a copy of their transcript for their amendments. A thematic coding system was developed. In analysis, themes emerged from the interviews, and theory was developed from them, rather than being tested by a pre-structured hypothesis (Strauss and Corbin, 1998). In reporting findings, identities were altered to maintain confidentiality.

Each interviewee was asked to talk about her experiences of working with women patients who self-cut, her own role in their care, her feelings and understandings about what was going on for the patient, for herself and the roles and responses of colleagues within the multi-disciplinary team. Issues around the nurses' needs, preparation and support for this work, were explored (Doy, 1995).

Interviewees used a range of words to describe the self-injuring behaviours of women:

> Superficially cutting ... ranging to cutting two to three inch cuts which require suturing. (Linda)

> A lot of women ... do mainly just scratch ... (Debbie)

> The cuts can get deeper and deeper and it's ... a ritual. (Bea)

The depth, the strength and the type of self-cutting were variously described as being on a continuum from picking and scraping, through scratching to gouging. These nurses' use of this vocabulary of self-cutting in discussing their relationship with the patient and care planning indicated how they understood and responded to these particular women patients.

Many means, usually everyday, accessible objects, have been reported as used by women to self-injure, including coins, fingernails, broken glass, razors, scissors, sharp surfaces, forks, self-biting and breaking bones (Doy, 1995; Pembroke, 1994). In the nurses' accounts, the desperation of the woman patient is clear. Reah's comments (below) underline the woman's need to know that she always has some available implement to cut with. Paradoxically, attempts to control or contain the self-injuring behaviour may serve to heighten her sense of powerlessness, leading to an escalation in self-cutting and attempts to secure objects for self-injury.

> She even took the insides out of Biros, the lead out of pencils, if she could get hold of them, and the plastic from the petals on the

Christmas tree lights. We had to keep searching her. The more we found, the more desperate she seemed to become, and anything she got hold of she'd use, even her bra (to attempt to strangle herself). (Reah)

The repetitiveness of the damaging actions is also conveyed:

Forks ... so that they have just scraped again and again and that they self-harm in the end, and they'd done it so many times ... so often. (Kate)

The literature reveals common themes underlying self-cutting behaviour. Malon and Beradi (1987) suggest that the trigger is often in perceiving the likelihood of separation, rejection or frustration. There is frequently an articulation of feelings of overwhelming tension and apprehension. Feelings of chaos, loss of control or emptiness spiral, anxiety builds, and a sense of unreality, void and, especially, depersonalization may be described.

Why do women injure themselves?

Four main themes regarding motivation for deliberate self-injury emerge from experiential and other empirical research evidence.

The first concerns handling and expressing feelings, including euphoria, easing tension or relief of anger. Many women who self-injure have great rage which they are afraid to express outwardly and so injure themselves as a way of venting these feelings (Favazza, 1989, 1996; Miller, 1994; Smith et al., 1998). Self-injury may also be motivated by a need for higher levels of stimulation. Adults who were repeatedly traumatized as children may find it difficult to return to a 'normal' baseline level of arousal and need crisis behaviour (Favazza, 1989, 1996).

A second motivational theme is that of escaping numbness and of needing to feel that one exists, and escaping from emptiness, depression and feelings of unreality (Favazza, 1989; 1996; Smith et al., 1998).

A third theme is that of obtaining or maintaining a sense of control over the behaviour of other people and over one's own body (Favazza, 1989; 1996). This is most often presumed by those working with women who self-injure and also misinterpreted as attention-seeking (Allen, 1995). For such women, successfully communicating feelings is often impossible in other media than 'writing the body', which may appear to be their only way to signal distress and bring some sense of control.

A fourth theme, relating to women who have been abused, is that such injury generates a way to continue an abusive pattern and to punish themselves when they carry beliefs of self-guilt and blame. Smith et al. (1998) argue that the parts of the body that are cut may be those areas that were attractive to the abuser.

All four themes include both psychosocial and psychodynamic factors especially relating to troubled relationships in the early formative childhood years. Ways in which these women have learned to cope at times of distress and family role-modelling in dealing with feelings, problems and relationships may also contribute (Burstow, 1992; 1998; Smith et al., 1998). Through these, self-injury may come to be seen as the medium of choice, or the only means, to communicate, vent feelings and signal being alive when feeling out of contact with oneself and consequently out of control (Burstow, 1992).

All psychoanalytic theorists trace distress and disruptive behaviour in adult life back to central traumas in childhood (Bowlby, 1971, 1975, 1980; Winnicott, 1964; 1986). For Bowlby, it relates to insecure attachments and the effect of losses and separation. For Winnicott, it is the effect of lacking a sense of being understood and secure which leads to the child and, later, the adult woman, feeling uncontained and, therefore, chaotic and lacking in control.

It may also be argued that women in particular are additionally confined to modes of communication permitted within patriarchal discourses, illustrated in this survivor account:

As little girls, we are taught to be ladylike and bite our lip. Little boys are encouraged to shout and let off steam. This conditioning stays with us in adulthood ... Personally, when I've seen the blood run I've felt relieved and purged. The stress recedes and I've felt as though I am back in control of my mind. Once more I have deflected those emotions and painful memories. ('Maggie', in Pembroke, 1994: p. 14)

Feminist theorists such as Burstow (1992) suggest that, unlike men, as women are not socialized to express violence externally, they tend to vent their rage on themselves. An effective therapeutic approach to self-injuring might therefore be expected to counter experiences of being silenced.

Therapeutic approaches to working with women who self-injure

The traditional medical model approach has tended to diminish the self-injuring woman as attention-seeking and therefore less deserving of treatment than men; this arguably manifests patriarchal 'binary' thinking (Cixous, in Moi, 1985).

Traditional treatment approaches – for example, physical interventions such as electroconvulsive therapy, and neuroleptic medication – are often experienced by patients as punitive, and so likely to increase anxiety and the need to cut (Pembroke, 1994; Smith et al., 1998). Such approaches concentrate more on symptom management than on working with inner need.

In contrast, Winnicott emphasizes the importance of treatment being based on a helping relationship, to counteract earlier disturbances in emotional development, thus 'enabling the patient's emotional development to go ahead where it was held up' (Winnicott, 1971: p. 157). The need for such a helping or therapeutic nurse–patient relationship is amplified in the stories of survivors and service users who have self-injured (Dace et al., 1998; Pembroke, 1994) and highlighted by all nurse interviewees in the author's research. They were clear that a caring environment and sensitivity of response by the nurse were essential for creating a climate of trust, change and a therapeutic space where the patient could explore her feelings and be supported in cutting herself less or with less risk. How this works is described here:

> they feel safe in beginning to express their feelings. They learn new ways of coping with their feelings and having outlets for their feelings and become a bit more aware of what they're doing to themselves or why they are hurting themselves ... (Reah)

An appropriate therapeutic approach depends on the value system and perception of the meaning of deliberate self-injury held by the helper. A key focus for the woman is to find her voice and be heard through developing a relationship which can encourage sensitivity and making sense of the layers of meaning underlying self-injuring activities. This is aptly illustrated as follows:

> I suppose I recognize more that it's not about looking at the presenting symptom, it's much more about looking at what went on behind

that symptom, and why they needed to feel that was the only way there was of expressing what it was like for them ... (Linda)

An empathic approach therefore emphasizes therapies such as art, photography, music and poetry, giving positive value to the expression of feelings and experiences and using media other than words (Smith et al., 1998).

Empowering the woman patient is central to an appropriate therapeutic approach (Burstow, 1992). This emphasizes support and consistency in setting limits and exploring alternative strategies for managing feelings, issues of control and coping. Repositioning the woman as a speaking (and heard) subject is integral to the therapeutic alliance and to deconstructing power imbalances. This may be a difficult process; so structured therapeutic interventions include relaxation or distraction strategies to reduce any build up of tension (Martinson, 1998; Smith et al., 1998). Minimizing the harm caused by self-cutting, reducing the number of times cutting is used or the depth of wounds incurred, may provide a realistic and self-controlling way for many women to feel less overwhelmed and to move forward therapeutically (Martinson, 1998; Smith et al., 1998). This requires an assertive, empowered helper who can negotiate the therapeutic programme with the woman, who understands the complexity of managing risk while supporting the patient in gaining a manageable level of personal responsibility. Structured psychotherapies, working to build self-esteem and challenge negative beliefs and thinking patterns, also provide successful and appropriate therapeutic approaches.

For many women, making contact with others who self-cut, to share understandings and reduce isolation, is vital (Martinson, 1998; Pembroke, 1992; Smith et al., 1998). Self-help groups, crisis telephone lines (such as the Bristol Crisis Service for Women referred to earlier) and survivor projects offer women who self-injure the chance to share their experiences with others with similar experiences.

All these examples provide elements of a therapeutic approach which establishes a process within which the woman can begin to learn about her feelings and be herself. This also involves supporting the patient to challenge or deconstruct a psychosocial life script within which self-injury is one of a few options. Working with these women may be draining, lengthy and frustrating. This approach therefore requires that the nurse-helper herself be empowered, with access to a framework of support and supervision within which she can offload and reflect on her practice and relationship with the patient. A therapeutic approach that neglects such support for therapists will be more likely to provide an environment in which stress and burnout may develop (Doy, 1995).

The author's research and other evidence suggest that an emerging 'empathic discourse' can usefully inform the therapeutic relationship to facilitate the woman who is self-injuring to 'reposition' herself by being heard as the speaking subject, to change and, at the very least, to hurt herself with less harm (Doy, 1995). There is clearly a continuing feminist task to raise awareness and understanding of the experience of the self-injuring woman and of the experience, qualities and skills required by nurses and other helpers. An informed, empathic and interdisciplinary therapeutic approach should continue to develop. The wounds from deliberate self-injury are both physical and emotional. Understanding the complex dynamics and meanings in self-cutting is essential if health and social care services, the friends and families of women who self-cut and the wider society, are to respond appropriately to this important aspect of women's health and distress.

Further reading

Favazza, A.R., *Bodies under Siege: Self-Mutilation and Body Modification in Culture and Psychiatry*, 2nd edn (Baltimore: The Johns Hopkins University Press, 1996).

Miller, D., *Women Who Hurt Themselves: A Book of Hope and Understanding* (New York: Basic Books, 1994).

Pembroke, L. (ed.), *Self-Harm: Perspectives from Personal Experience* (London: Survivors Speak Out, 1994).

Smith, G., Cox, D. and Saradjian, J., *Women and Self-Harm* (London: The Woman's Press, 1998).

4
Women, Drugs and Alcohol

Jan Keene

Introduction

While it is clear that both drug misuse and alcohol misuse have increased among women (OPCS, 1992), creating problems for their health, women still lack support from helping agencies (DAWN, 1994; Waterson and Ettore, 1989). This chapter begins with a brief examination of the nature of drug and alcohol misuse which considers the different treatment perspectives and reviews the research evidence. As most of the existing literature does not consider gender issues, the second section examines specifically what the published work can contribute to understanding the nature of women's drug and alcohol problems. It does so by highlighting the social and psychological issues which underlie female alcohol and drug misuse, the factors which constrain its solutions and the implications for developing service provision.

A major difficulty in dealing with the complexity of substance misuse problems arises from the commonly held view of misuse as creating homogeneous and universal problems connected to dependency or addiction (Keene, 1997). This is exacerbated by the particular focus of existing research on this subject, which strongly emphasizes the consequences for pregnancy, children and child abuse, and parenting. At its most narrow, the public debate concentrates on serious alcohol abuse or the effects of heroin on pregnant women (see, for example, Jacob, 1986; Mertin, Harmer and Sanderson, 1999; Orford and Vellman, 1996; Priest, 1990).

Furthermore, women may be subject to a double standard concerning substance misuse; conventional interpretations often ignore the 'gendering' of substance misuse and women's social and political positions (Henderson 1999; Waterson and Ettore, 1989). Keil (1978), for example, presented evidence that women were more likely to use alcohol to resolve sex role conflicts. Later research identifying the specific events which cause substance misuse in women rather than men (Cook and Allen, 1984; Kent, 1989; Robinson, 1988) focused on how the social context of women's drinking is related to their gender.

An understanding of women's substance use and misuse should be placed in the context of a comprehensive sociological analysis of women's place in society. Such an analysis suggests that typical stereotypes of women in Western society shed light on the social and political problems of women who attempt to seek help or to rehabilitate themselves. For example, the characterization of female drug misusers as weak, passive and, usually, pathological and maladaptive as individuals (Ettore, 1992; Henderson, 1999; Oppenheimer, 1994) produces problems for such women in managing their everyday social relationships. It also contributes to their difficulties when women attempt to get help for child care or employment.

In addition, women seeking help or treatment for substance misuse, or other social and health problems, may find the route impeded by attitudes emanating from professional value bases rooted in the need for change, rather than for psychosocial maintenance (Keene, 2001). Taylor (1994) has also demonstrated that much psychiatric and medical literature describes women as morally deficient and as more deviant than men. The woman who misuses drugs and alcohol is seen as trying to adopt aspects of the male stereotype and therefore rejecting the dominant social conception of femininity imposed on women (Zimmer-Hofler and Dobler-Mikola, 1992).

Much information about women was sparse or distorted until the 1990s (Oppenheimer, 1994), when reviews such as Plant's (1990) of women's alcohol use and Ettore's (1992), overview of substance misuse among women began to explore the gender issues inherent in women's substance use and related problems.

In considering the particular needs of women misusing alcohol and drugs, this chapter attempts to avoid previous pitfalls (Oppenheimer, 1994) by shifting the focus more widely than just the rights of the foetus and the needs of children, to the gender-specific needs for care. Such needs often arise from psychological and social differences such as childhood abuse or increased vulnerability to violence and intimidation as adults.

Alcohol and drug misuse: a complex range of problems

From an international perspective, substance misuse has expanded dramatically, through both the greatly increased use of established drugs, and also the appearance of newer, more harmful patterns of use (World Health Organization Expert Committee, 1989). For Britain, the evidence demonstrates repeatedly how the widespread use of alcohol is a major cause of illness and is closely associated with violence and criminal behaviour among a small proportion of drinkers (Plant, 1990). In addition, with the wider use of illegal drugs, there is evidence of more harmful use among a minority of users (Strang and Gossop, 1994). However, both alcohol and drug misuse should be viewed within a wider context of substantial recreational or non-problematic drug misuse (Keene, 1997).

While most research concentrates on dependent or addicted substance misuse, recent work indicates that problematic substance misuse varies over the life course, rather than a uniform sequence of heavy use leading to addiction, followed by treatment and abstinence (Keene, 1997; Lindstrom, 1992; Moos et al., 1990). Substance use and problematic use varies over time, with irregular periods of controlled use and uncontrolled or chaotic use. The latter is often associated with mental health or psychological problems, crisis, stress or changes in relationships and social group (Najavits et al., 1997). At such times drug and alcohol misuse may increase and dependency and other problems also accumulate.

The place of treatment in such a long-term pattern of misuse is unclear. It may bring about no more than a temporary spell of abstinence or controlled use following a particularly severe period of substance misuse. Support available at times of stress may relieve problems of increasing misuse; if available after treatment, such support may reduce the possibility of relapse.

Women's substance misuse, whether dependent or not, has been found to be strongly associated with psychological and social problems (DAWN, 1994; Ettore, 1992; Galaif et al., 1999; Merton et al., 1999; Oppenheimer, 1994). These contribute to the development and the maintenance of misuse and dependency and related problems. They also help prevent their resolution.

Thus, early childhood abuse and psychological problems can lead to women using drugs and alcohol to cope or to their self-medicating. However, such drug and alcohol use, which may lead, for example, to criminality or dependency, bring their own problems which then compound the issues to be tackled.

This chapter is not concerned with women who use alcohol and drugs in recreational or non-problematic ways, but neither is it limited to those who are dependent or addicted. Its focus is on all women whose substance use becomes problematic at various times over their lives, examining the causes of these problems and the obstacles to their solution.

Treatment and the development of more complex solutions

It is commonly assumed that the main problem associated with drug and alcohol use is misuse-related dependency. Dependency is viewed as an illness or psychological problem rather than as a solution to other problems. Therefore, the response is seen as treatment of such dependency, whether medical, psychological or psychotherapeutic. However, recent research evidence suggests that drug-related health and social issues may be equally, if not more, important targets for action (Henderson, 1999; Moos et al., 1990; SCODA, 1997; Thom and Green, 1996).

Within the treatment field, there are four main treatment perspectives of dependency: the cognitive behavioural approach; the medical or physiological approach; the disease or Twelve Step model; and the Dependence Syndrome (Edwards; 1988; 1989). The cognitive behavioural approach utilizes psychological methods from social learning theory and cognitive psychology to change dependent or risky behaviours: this is termed 'controlled drinking' for alcohol problems and 'harm minimization' for drug problems. The medical or physiological approach focuses on physical addiction and provides withdrawal programmes. The Twelve Step disease model of Alcoholics Anonymous and Narcotics Anonymous uses a different understanding of dependency, as a disease of the whole person, and provides an intensive therapeutic recovery programme. The Dependence Syndrome is a combination of psychological, medical and social perspectives. All four models have been adapted for both drugs and alcohol dependency but none explicitly addresses gender differences.

However, outcome researchers in the substance misuse field have been unable to distinguish between these four models in terms of effectiveness in reducing severity of dependence and/or drinking behaviour. Each model results in a successful treatment outcome for between a third and a half of cases (Lindstrom, 1992). In the light of this information, researchers have tried, but failed, to identify individual or personality characteristics which predispose some people to do better with particular treatments (Lindstrom, 1992; Moos et al., 1990).

Indeed, some research suggests that some non-treatment methods (pragmatic helping tools) may be more successful than treatment models. These successful methods are concerned more with social factors and improved social functioning, which prove significant in terms of pre-treatment characteristics and treatment outcome (Hodgson, 1994; Lindstrom, 1992).

This work has led to an interest in the interactive effects of different treatment models and a wide range of individual and social variables. Research indicates that, although specific treatment variables may be significant for immediate behaviour change, many other variables mediate treatment effects. This is further complicated by variables influencing maintenance of change at follow-up, such as personal and social functioning (Lindstrom, 1992; Moos et al., 1990).

Such academic controversy about the accuracy and effectiveness of treatment models is reflected in contemporary professional debates about appropriate assessment criteria and psychological or social interventions between psychologists, health professionals, social workers and specialist counsellors.

These debates may have a serious impact on service provision in limiting inter-professional communication and collaboration, and reducing the chances of cohesive and comprehensive help for people with substance misuse problems. They therefore have additional, important implications for our understanding of development of substance misuse among women and therefore, also, of gender-specific solutions.

Gender differences

The research findings discussed above are directly relevant to understanding drug and alcohol misuse amongst women because psychological and social factors significant in developing and maintaining drug and alcohol problems may well be gender-specific (DAWN, 1994; Ellenwood et al., 1966; Ettore, 1992; Ladwig and Anderson, 1989; Oppenheimer, 1994; Nelson-Zlupko et al., 1995). Psychological problems include those arising from early childhood abuse and abusive adult relationships. Therefore depression, anxiety and psychopathology are high among this group (Zlupko et al., 1995). Social problems include co-dependency, prostitution and associated criminal lifestyles where women may be particularly vulnerable (Taylor, 1994).

Similarly, if personal and social functioning are the critical factors in recovery, these are likely to be related to the particular psychological problems and social factors which influence a woman's life (Ladwig and Anderson, 1989; Merton, 1999).

However, such research has not specifically examined the nature of gender differences for women (Ettore, 1992) and neither has research in the treatment field. Nevertheless, recent studies of the needs of women and the appropriateness of gender-specific service provision (for example, Thom and Green, 1996) indicate that attitudes towards women are slowly beginning to change. It is now well established that men and women differ not only in their reasons for misusing alcohol and drugs, but also in different patterns of misuse and their reasons for relapse (Ettore, 1992; Ladwig and Anderson, 1989). For alcohol, there is now a substantial body of evidence that women drink less than men, are likely to experience fewer alcohol-related harms and are involved less in alcohol-related crime (DAWN, 1994; Plant, 1990) Such gender differences are found internationally (Thom and Green, 1996). Nevertheless, drinking is seen as appropriate for men but not for women who, when heavy drinkers, are still widely regarded as flawed and degenerate (Ellenwood et al., 1966; Jefferies, 1983; Kent, 1989; Robinson, 1988; Wolfson and Murray, 1986), especially in relation to child-bearing and child care (Ettore, 1989; Nelson-Zlupko et al., 1995). Clearly, therefore, the research evidence is partial and this limitation must be borne in mind in the following analysis.

Psychological problems

The great majority of women with drug or alcohol problems use these substances to counter negative states rather than to enhance positive states (Rosenbaum, 1981). Such women frequently have a history of sexual or physical abuse (Ladwig and Anderson, 1989; Merton et al., 1999; Wolfson and Murray, 1986). There is a strong tendency for women to use sedative drugs rather than stimulants or prescribed drugs (Keene, 1997). Although many of these women are diagnosed as having high levels of psychopathology before and after treatment, requiring treatment earlier than men, they do make more attempts to stop their misuse (Nelson-Zlupko et al., 1995). While we know little about the specific psychological problems associated with drug and alcohol misuse, there is a clear indication that this would be a fruitful area of research.

Social problems

Women who misuse drugs commonly have a relationship with male partners who are also misusers of drugs and/or alcohol and who are often in control of supply, the amount and the means of consumption (Gordon and Barrett, 1993; Keene, 1997; Rosenbaum, 1981). There is a well-documented, close relationship between alcohol and drug misuse and crime, for both men and women (Rosenbaum, 1981; Strang and Gossop, 1994). Financing addiction is a prime motivation of criminal behaviour, with drug-related crime accounting for a high proportion of offences (Strang and Gossop, 1994; Taylor, 1993). The patterns of criminal behaviour are, however, quite different for men and women. Shoplifting, fraud, forgery and, particularly, prostitution are most frequent for women, with a discernible sequence beginning with shoplifting (Hammersley et al., 1990). This activity becomes much more risky as the women become known to store detectives. There are also limitations to the resort to fraud. Although prostitution is seen by these women as a last resort (Rosenbaum, 1981; Taylor, 1993), estimates indicate that between 40 per cent and 70 per cent of female addicts have resorted to it (Goldstein, 1979; Weisberg, 1985; Wolfson and Murray, 1986). Research suggests a circularity in this phenomenon, with women more often misusing drugs to face the ordeal of prostitution from which the financial rewards lead to an escalating dependency, requiring them to continue as prostitutes (Taylor, 1994; Weisberg, 1985).

While there is not the evidence to say what proportion of women are affected, it is clear that the use of illegal drugs, and the activities which pay for it, can lead to women being drawn into the criminal world, where the drug subculture generates a caricature of chauvinistic male–female relations, characterized by a high incidence of sexual abuse and violence (Ettore, 1989; James, 1976; Jefferies, 1983; Najavits et al., 1997).

Pregnant drug misusers

As noted earlier, pregnancy and child care issues have dominated the attention of researchers and policy-makers (SCODA, 1997) This may reflect women's role as the bearers of children and the expectation of their prime responsibility for child care.

Therapists and social workers concerned with women may view pregnancy as providing an opportunity for their clients to cut down on drugs or abstain, give up their previous lifestyle and take up new responsibilities (Norman-Bruce and Kearney, 1990; Nelson-Zlupko et al., 1995). Here, the nature of agency support can be clearly defined. In contrast, doctors and paediatricians frequently believe that pregnancy creates new difficulties (Hogg, 1989). They prefer to stabilize the pregnant woman, using heroin or methadone on a continuous programme, to help her cope more effectively with the baby (Hogg, 1989; SCODA, 1997).

Underlying these differing perspectives is the very difficult issue of maternal versus foetal rights (Bainham, 1998; Gardner, 1992). Recent UK legislation, notably the Children Act 1989 (see also Department of Health, 1991), ensures that a care order may be based on presumed risk, even where harm cannot be established (Bainham, 1998). In contrast, the Standing Conference on Drug and Alcohol Abuse (SCODA) guidelines (1997) state that evidence of substance misuse is not, in itself, evidence that drug-taking mothers are less likely to be adequate parents. Even where chaotic misuse is a possible source of potential danger to the foetus and to the child, these guidelines state that support and encouragement should be given to stabilize misuse to minimize harm rather than to enforce abstinence and withdrawal. Again, there is clearly much controversy in this area.

Parental alcohol and drug misuse

Women alcohol and drug misusers are more likely to have responsibility for dependent children than their male counterparts. There is a growing awareness of the need to resolve conflicts between providing help for drinking and drug-using parents and child care issues. This is reflected in training which encourages drug workers and child care social workers to collaborate and consider the welfare of the parent and child in tandem. While the Children Act gives opportunities for agencies to gain support for clients with children (Department of Health, 1991), Norman-Bruce and Kearney (1990) argue that drug workers need training in child protection. Tracey and Farkas (1994), in America, also argue that practitioners need to be trained for working with children in families with substance misuse. In contrast, Cohen (1990) highlights the problems for social workers trying to deal with drug misuse problems.

There are considerable variations between countries in the Western world in the attitudes and policies concerning parents and substance misuse. In some countries there is a general tolerance of such parents, while others take a much more restrictive view (SCODA, 1997; Waterson and Ettore, 1989; Zimmer-Hofler and Dobler-Mikola, 1992).

This is further complicated by the existence of differing priorities of those professionals dealing with child welfare and those whose work is directed towards adults (SCODA, 1997). In general, parental substance misuse is regarded as having deleterious consequences for dependent children, without considering the differences in types of effects and risks associated with different patterns of drug and alcohol use.

Developing appropriate service provision for women

The implications of this research for policy and practice can be considered in four areas. 1) There are problems surrounding lack of information and stereotypical views of women's substance misuse, and the ways to combat these problems through education and information for clients and training for professionals. 2) This problem of lack of information is reflected in narrow and specialized assessments that are determined by theories of dependency rather than being needs-led (Keene, 1997; Sullivan et al., 1992). The solution, therefore, can be seen in more comprehensive assessments that focus on psychological and social needs rather than only on narrower definitions of treatment issues. 3) Service provision for women needs to be adapted to deal with underlying psychological problems and social context of substance misuse. 4) The research indicates that assessments and resulting interventions will be more effective if they are aimed at the psychological and social problems which underpin and maintain dependency, as well as at the treatment of dependency (Buckley and Bigelow, 1992; Sullivan et al., 1992; Sullivan and Hartmann, 1994). If psychological and social problems are relevant in both the development of dependency and its cure, this necessitates taking gender differences into account in the development of policy and practice.

Information-giving

As with many policy and practice initiatives, it is important to ensure that research evidence is relayed to clients and patients as well as professionals, to enable the development of common understandings of assessments and effective solutions to problems. The review of research indicates that professionals may not be aware of the implications of gender differences for women (Adams, 1999; SCODA, 1997; Nelson-Zlupko et al., 1995).

In addition, there is a need for accurate factual information concerning the different effects of types of alcohol and drug misuse on the foetus throughout pregnancy. As this is an area of active research, regular updating of accessible information is imperative to enable pregnant women, mothers and, for that matter, professionals make informed decisions.

Similarly, information needs to be provided on which types of alcohol and drug-misuse are most likely to lead to abuse or neglect, not only for women's dependent substance misuse, but also for women's chaotic, unstable use without social support.

Service development

There is evidence to demonstrate that, where a comprehensive assessment of psychological and social factors is carried out, the resulting intervention will be more effective. One example would be an interdisciplinary team approach to treatment of drug dependence and associated disorders, with the focus of treatment on identifying high-risk and other problem situations, training in coping skills to handle those situations, developing insight and enhancing motivation. Buckley and Bigelow's (1992) example of an interdisciplinary service incorporating mental health, probation, social and housing agencies as well as drug and alcohol treatment agencies suggests that such comprehensive service provision is more cost-effective than fragmentary service provision. Sullivan et al. (1992; 1994) suggest that professionals should tackle drug and alcohol use by focusing on community functioning and social rehabilitation and, in this way, help prevent relapse. This is particularly relevant for women where gender-specific social factors, such as support for child care, influence how treatment gains are maintained.

The issues related to social support are particularly relevant for substance-misusing parents, indicating that parental training should be aimed at strengthening informal support networks for child care as well as parenting skills (SCODA, 1997). Supportive family and friends have been shown to be crucially important here (Adams, 1999; Moos et al., 1990). In addition, formal support for child care is required during periods of treatment and relapse. While there are many potential developments in service provision, based on dealing with psychological and social problems, the cardinal requirement is that women should feel safe to ask for help and support without fear of losing their children (Adams, 1999; Hogg, 1989; Keene, 1997). This can best be achieved where there are clear and unequivocal guidelines for both professionals and clients about the limits of acceptable child care and the support available when necessary (Hogg, 1989; SCODA, 1997). To be effective it is essential that this is seen to be provided, particularly in periods of crisis, on a continual basis rather than being linked to 'treatment success' (SCODA, 1997).

Gender-specific treatment programmes

Treatment interventions tailored to women's needs are rare (Adams, 1999; Oppenheimer, 1994; Nelson-Zlupko et al., 1995). Such programmes must give full attention to the identification of psychological problems and the negative emotions that contribute to alcohol and drug misuse or lead to relapse (Keene, 1997). They need to establish personal autonomy and ways of dealing with co-dependence (Ladwig and Anderson, 1989). There is a specific need to provide treatment and support for such problems as depression, anorexia and bulimia (Ladwig and Anderson, 1989).

Providing a safe (female-only) therapeutic environment with professional expertise available is also important, but may raise problems if, for example, it is difficult to find people to care for children (Adams, 1999; Stewart, 1987).

Confronting the occurrence of prostitution, abuse and criminal connections is also often necessary. This requires harm-minimization and protection for those women who wish to remove themselves from the criminal subculture, where they may be victimized and intimidated (Henderson, 1999; Zimmer-Hofler and Dobler-Mikola, 1992; Nelson-Zlupko et al., 1995). For those women who wish to remain as prostitutes, practical support and help leading to risk management and safe working is of great importance (Goldstein, 1979; James, 1976). This should, perhaps, go hand in hand with the attempt to encourage women's autonomy in heterosexual relationships, and their assertiveness, with due regard to any dangers for them in changing the dynamics of their relationships.

Conclusion

This brief analysis has indicated the types of problems that arise for women who misuse alcohol and drugs, and which may help maintain misuse and cause relapse. As the research suggests, the importance of psychological and social issues especially gender-specific in these processes will have particular implications for women. They should lead to less over-concentration on the treatment of substance dependency in favour of more broad-based assessments and, therefore, a more comprehensive range of interventions.

In conclusion, it is necessary not only to offer safe gender-specific treatment for dependency but also to tackle both the gender-specific psychological problems that cause the substance misuse and the social problems that maintain it. Treatment services and gender-specific programmes therefore need to focus more on the psychological problems which underpin much female addiction, such as depression, eating disorders and co-dependence. In addition, protection, social support, education and employment opportunities are necessary to offer women empowering alternatives. The overall aim of services for women must be to break the cycle of emotional and financial dependency rather than narrowly attending to substance dependency.

Further reading

Ettore, B., *Women and Substance Use* (Basingstoke: Macmillan, 1992).

Keene, J., *Clients with Complex Needs: Interprofessional Practice* (Oxford: Blackwell Science, 2001).

Plant, M., *Women and Alcohol: A Review of the International Literature on Use of Alcohol by Females* (Geneva: World Health Organization, 1990).

SCODA, *Drug-Using Parents: Policy Guidelines for Inter-Agency Working* (London LGA Publications, 1997).

5
Beyond Health and Beauty: A Critical Perspective on Fitness Culture

Roberta Sassatelli

As more women are invited to take up exercise as a way to keep healthy, fitness training has rapidly become their principal path into physical activity. A critical appraisal of fitness helps to understand where lines may be drawn between healthy and unhealthy practices, as ideals drawn on by women engaging in fitness, which can be shown to go well beyond – and possibly against – technical and traditional notions of health. This chapter therefore focuses on the meanings women associate with their fitness training. These meanings are explored together with expert discourse on fitness, to examine the body ideal promoted by keep-fit culture, its relations with health and beauty and the broader cultural values underpinning women's efforts in the gym.

Expert discourse on fitness training, whether academic or commercial, states that physical exercise is good for the body, boosting strength and energy and helping prevent illnesses. Popular fitness magazines are particularly keen to portray exercise in the gym as a panacea which not only fosters a contemporary version of beauty – 'correcting wrong postures', 'getting rid of excessive fat', 'toning muscles' – but also produces health – 'lowering cholesterol', 'strengthening the heart', 'preventing osteoporosis'. Medical discourse itself increasingly attributes both preventive and therapeutic qualities to physical activity. In turn 'good physical fitness' is portrayed, even by official European Union documents, as 'an indispensable component of overall well-being' (Oja and Tuxworth, 1995: p. 6). However, if we use a sociological approach to think about fitness training, we cannot then view it merely in terms of taken-for-granted, objective, physical or physiological benefits. This is so, first, because there is little agreement even among the most accredited medical experts, whose prescriptions vary widely as to quantity, frequency and quality of 'healthy' physical activity (Glassner, 1992; Shephard, 1995; Solomon, 1984). And second, a sociologist also needs to examine the history of different ways in which health and physical exercise have come to be related (Berryman, 1992), the meanings that fitness participants associate with their practices and the broader social values promoted by fitness culture.

Fitness culture has attracted much interest, especially from recent Marxist-feminist thought, in examining gender differences and the physical ideals prized within some of the most noticeable techniques, such as aerobics and body-building. Usually, their aim is to expose the extent to which participants incorporate oppressive forms of femininity. The success of aerobics videos, for example, has been interpreted as evidence that women are still victims of a patriarchal regime which obliges them to worry about their appearance, training to the exclusive advantage of the male gaze, so reproducing an uncompromising, commercially promoted body ideal (Weitz and Dinnerstein, 1998). Others portray aerobics as a form of female-dominated physical activity which segregates women, fails to promote self-acceptance and focuses on fat in ways reflecting the obsessions which haunt women with eating disorders (Lloyd, 1996; Maguire and Mansfield, 1998). Body-building, in turn, has been seen as creating a subculture which reproduces a type of femininity which is all too conspicuously oppositional to the conventionally masculine, rather than subverting the dichotomy. Female body-builders seem to challenge gender dichotomies, yet, in competitions, must resort to conventional feminine postures, make-up and hair styles (Lowe, 1998; Mansfield and McGinn, 1993).

The approach adopted in this chapter takes a different perspective from an exclusive emphasis on how physical activity may be used to establish domination, by accepting that fitness training can provide both improved body functionality and individual self-esteem. Some feminists have expressed doubts about condemning fitness training. Markula (1995), amongst others, suggests that such practices can generate critical voices with the potential to alter the course of dominant practices. Her ethnographic study of US female 'aerobicizers' shows that women 'struggle to obtain the ideal body, but they also find their battle ridiculous' (Markula, 1995: 424). She underlines the gender ambivalence in aerobics' promotion of curvaceous muscularity, thus creating a hybrid feminine image which combines the traditional image with a stronger, androgynous one. Developing Markula's findings, this chapter suggests fitness training is an ambivalent phenomenon, a social practice which both offers women new capacities and knowledge and also secures its own reproduction by bestowing normative force to these capacities and knowledge. Likewise, fitness cannot be said to be wholly healthy. Rather it promotes its own version of health.

To appreciate this entails understanding meanings attributed to fitness by regular exercisers and experts. It is not enough to observe how fitness training is portrayed in the media or to draw on survey data. We need an approach such as ethnography (Hammersley and Atkinson, 1983) to observe how interactions are conducted 'on the ground' within fitness gyms. In this way the researcher can learn what manners, practices and values are important for the different actors involved, collecting an array of different participants' voices by conducting formal and informal interviews.

This chapter draws on an ethnographic project conducted in Italy from 1994 to 1995 (Sassatelli, 2000). Two very different fitness gyms, constituting the two extreme poles of fitness offered within one middle-class neighbourhood, were studied for over six months to identify what may be considered as 'typical' of keep-fit culture (Yin, 1989). This chapter can claim only to interpret meanings within a specific (Italian) context, but does attempt to develop some analytical generalization of the distinctive body ideal which fitness training may crystallize. The following discussion draws on the analysis of all relevant ethnographic sources collected: field notes from participant observation, informal interviews with clients, trainers and managers, and in-depth interviews with clients. It also draws on the analysis of a wide selection of expert discourse on gymnastics including a sample of manuals covering different types of exercise, body objectives and target groups, and all Italian periodical publications on fitness from 1994 to 1996. Participants' real names have been changed to protect confidentiality, while words or phrases in quotes draw faithfully from interviews, conversations and fieldnotes.

Striving for fitness

Fitness gyms involve a variety of exercise techniques, ranging from aerobic and anaerobic machine training to different classes such as aerobics, step, stretching, yoga and tai chi. As suggested by fitness manuals and magazines, these gyms also place emphasis on 'well-being' or 'feeling better'. In contrast with traditional sports, fitness training officially has nothing to do with a struggle for superiority, appearing as a perfect example of what Bourdieu (1978: p. 839) defined as 'health-oriented sports': physical activities which 'do not offer any competitive satisfaction'. Fitness manuals invite prospective gym-goers 'to avoid competition with other participants', stressing that 'there will be no prize for that person who becomes tall, slim, slender before anyone else'. During the many different lessons I witnessed, the instructors often stigmatized competition. They insisted to clients that there be 'no challenge amongst' participants, not to 'check what others are able to do' and that 'everyone' had to concentrate on herself.

This does not demand the denial of all challenges. Competition is replaced by self-challenge, a striving to better one's own exercise performances which, indeed, has been observed as prevalent in fitness discourses across the world (Amir, 1987; Morse, 1987/8). I repeatedly encountered trainers who incited clients to continue exercise, using images of combat. During a difficult step sequence, I learned that fat was 'burnt' and 'attacked'. Getting to the end of an aerobics class, I was invited, like all participants, to 'hold on, up to the breaking-point'. Machine-training also requires that each participant 'pushes to the limits of one's own strength'. In these exercise spaces, clients are asked to enter into a world where there is no competition with other participants. Everyone is none the less provided with an equivalent (not equal) body whose performances can and should be the object of continuous self-challenge.

This configuration yields two intertwined features of fitness training. Contrary to athletic sports, fitness gyms deny any scarcity – of desires, capacities, honours, and so on. This field of action, rather, generates a pluralistic abundance of non-competitive gratifications. The lack of challenge with external opponents or of getting one's achievements recognized in an official hierarchy, is replaced by novelty. As regular clients suggested, as exercise capacities improve, to continue training one needs ever newer incentives, techniques and trainers, as well as exploring more difficult activities. Similarly, all trainers and managers interviewed insisted that clients should consider their gym as a place where everyone has to find a 'personal' way of training by making the most of the array of techniques and novelties available. In the gym, the possibility of choosing among different techniques is concretely underlined in many practical ways: all techniques are easily accessible; their place on the timetable varies over the week; notices promote new techniques or machines. Above all, there is symbolic support for selecting and combining different techniques, by all being presented as sound, guaranteed alternatives for each other. Although different, in calling forth specific individual resources and physical qualities, the activities of a fitness gym are portrayed by trainers as 'equally good' and 'positive', effectively 'available' to each client to improve their bodies. The overall effect is to boost and tie clients' multifarious desires to a minimum common denominator. The better body promised by fitness is primarily a 'toned' body, full of 'energy' and 'power'.

Two different visions of fitness are therefore being simultaneously presented. On the one hand, we find a pluralistic vision of both exercise (it is 'not important what exercise you do, only that you do some') and physique ('no matter what size or shape you are, the thing is to get toned'). On the other, we find an abstract but strongly normative underlying common denominator; the fit body, available to 'everyone' who works for it. Amy, a part-time university student in her late twenties and a regular gym client, maintains that doing some keep-fit programme helps her appreciate the importance of a 'vigorous' body rather than fixating on 'appearances', and precisely because 'everyone can go [to the gym] and get these qualities', the fit body image embraces all.

The abstract body ideal reinforced by fitness training contrasts with the ideal promoted by body-building. Body-building was born as a 'popular', masculine search for strength realized through an aesthetic development of the muscles, in particular the upper body. It appeals to a 'morpho-structural' notion of the body which 'searches in forms for a sign of strength'. This contrasts with a 'functional' notion of the body, still relating to muscles but concerned with 'invisible', deep qualities like energy and resistance (Louveau, 1981: p. 305; see also Rabinbach, 1990; Vigarello, 1978) which inspire today's fitness culture.

The historian Park (1994: pp. 61–2) explains that 'Victorians tended to think of fitness in terms of biological adaptiveness' with athletes therefore 'often depicted as biologically superior males', whereas today 'fitness is often equated with muscle size, body contour, and/or the ability to sustain a 30-minute exercise bout'. Indeed, in my research I could observe that trainers and experts often suggest that muscles are 'involved in everything'; 'the more they are toned, the more they move with ease, and every single activity is turned into something less tiring'. In exploring the meanings associated with the fit body ideal, we see that this collates a number of different qualities such as energy, strength, resistance, agility, elasticity, vascular capacity, stamina. All of these portray the body as a basic resource for coping with the varied demands of everyday life. Fitness manuals, for example, often insist that a person in 'good physical form' can 'withstand fatigue for much longer than an unfit person', and, that 'there exists a direct relation between physical form, on the one hand, and intellectual vivacity and absence of nervous tension, on the other'.

Fitness, health and beauty

The fitness culture presents fitness training as aiming to augment the *universal utility* of the body, its capacity to face opportunities and accidents, as pure instrumentality with multifunctional utility. As pure instrumentality, the body is not just the instrument to carry out the exercise routine, but also, and more importantly, is the instrument of the self in the world. Thus a gym fan like Glenys, a middle-aged, part-time physiotherapist who wants to 'keep in good form', defines physical form as 'being more elastic, toned, feeling well, physically, with yourself. It is not like looking at oneself in the mirror and saying "Ah, I look good!" It is feeling oneself at ease with one's own body.' For Glenys, keeping oneself fit is not 'necessarily linked to health', but it 'helps facing whatever may happen to you' in ordinary life situations, like when 'you go shopping and if you carry five or six bags, if you have not exercised you feel it'.

These words address the particular contribution of the ideal of the fit body in bridging health and beauty, offering a new vision of both. As Goldstein (1992) suggests, expert discourse on fitness is different from official medical discourse, dominated by the 'Asclepius' model conceiving health as the result of specific interventions aiming to eliminate illness. Rather, fitness is inspired by an 'Igeia' model, where health is conceived as something everyone can acquire by living in harmony with nature and by following self-imposed routines to produce a particular kind of health – above all, vitality and energy. A popular gymnastic handbook appropriately entitled *Always Young* maintains that 'feeling good' is above all to 'be healthy and efficient': 'one can be strong, healthy, active and in love at any age'; thus the objective of fitness training is 'not only that of adding years to the lifespan, but rather that of adding some life to one's years'. Such a concept of health goes well beyond the absence of illness and what is now defined, even by the World Health Organization, as 'positive health'. The fitness concept is of a *healthy physical form*, or a 'general functional adequacy to withstand physical challenges without overstrain' (Oja and Tuxworth, 1995: p. 7). Such a body is an instrument whose internal functioning is to be stimulated for its utility in working for the subject in the world.

In Italian fitness gyms, stretching, soft techniques or varying combinations of dance, aerobics and weight exercises are more popular than straight aerobics. None the less the views of Morse on the beauty ideal of aerobics are relevant: namely, that the spread of aerobics meant that 'the once-masculine province of exercise' became 'part of commercial beauty culture' producing a 'new muscular femininity' (Morse, 1987/8: p. 23). Similarly, most fitness activities promote *well-toned forms* as the ideal figure (Markula, 1995).

Most women going to the gym tend to develop a particular aesthetic taste relating to the ideal body, inspired by functionality. Some more assiduous clients explain that people who work out manage to perform minor gestures of everyday life, 'picking something up' or 'bending' in a 'physically' and 'aesthetically more correct way for the muscles', with 'agility', without 'squatting', 'springing up' in the 'right way'. More generally, they claim that working out fosters 'a different way of relating to people' because you leave the gym 'with a certain way of walking', a certain body 'demeanour', 'standing straighter', feeling 'more oxygenated' and being 'more active'. The body's aerobic and anaerobic workout is both a means to obtain an ideal shape and also an intimate feature of that shape. Fitness, therefore, is also expressed aesthetically in a model of toned, compact body mass and well-defined curves indicating muscular energy. The aesthetics of functionality demand that the body be not large but strong, nimble and supple. Muscles, rather than bulk, must be strengthened, firmed and elongated.

To sum up, fitness experts and regular clients agree on an overlap between muscular efficiency, the rationalized movement of muscles and greater physical fitness. A fit body is the product of well-organized physical activity. This signifies an instrumental vision of the body kept active as an energy reserve to exploit in daily life. However, this energy emanates from a body shape which can be seen. Energy is not only an instrument to be used by the subject in the world, but an energetic *look* is also a crucial indicator of the subject's worth. The instrumentality of the body produced by fitness training becomes a meaningful value. A body with a well-defined outline, erect posture, more muscle and less fat is also appreciated as a 'sign' of the subject's energy, vitality and strength. If, as Foucault (1991b: pp. 137, 152) claims, a 'disciplined body is the prerequisite of an efficient gesture' and 'the only truly important ceremony is that of exercise', a body which has visibly incorporated exercise acquires ceremonial properties. A fit body, capable of sustaining a broad range of gestures, movements and exercises, tells us something about the subject. Although body language is not the object of working out in the gym, a fit body acquires symbolic value, hinting at a strong self, in control of herself.

Fitness and the modern self

Fitness enthusiasts appear to have declared war on fat: although working out can correct asymmetries, the ideal shape is first and foremost defined by a 'firm' and 'modelled' outline. The clients whom I interviewed all seemed to consider fat 'a dead weight', a useless and uncontrollable part of their bodies, full of 'toxins', a sign of 'old age', and a source of 'disease'. But pursuing this war was not merely material – moral values pulse beneath this materiality. Fitness is portrayed as a practice which makes women feel better through taking care of their bodies. Yet participants describe such 'taking care of the body' as a 'means' to 'keep the body functioning well' and to bring it 'under the control' of the self. Many stress that a functioning body full of 'positive energy' which can be 'exploited at its best' is 'just very useful' to the self in 'every social occasion'. Despite the emphasis on individual choice and a proclaimed pluralistic attitude, the legitimation of the gym is bound not only to a particular, normative vision of the body, but also to a particular, normative image of subjectivity.

Training in the gym is portrayed as not only rational, exact and effective; it is also 'right', 'correct' and 'virtuous'. Callan Pickney is an American trainer whose manuals are world-wide bestsellers, widely circulated in Italy. She says that physical exercise becomes part of our lives because 'nature needs a push' and that only we can 'take our lives in our hands', 'stop complaining' and 'get to work out'. In other words, recourse to the notion of nature provides a moral justification. Lisa, a young student from a lower-middle-class background explains that 'improving your external appearance', 'is not vanity' if it is the fruit of physical activity, if it is achieved 'by natural means, being careful what you do with your body'. Lisa's words echo the majority of clients: exercise is natural since it engages the body's intrinsic capacity for change, and training is 'work on your own body by your own body'. Most of these interviewees considered the use of the body's energy for the purposes of changing it as providing a moral emphasis, thereby giving fitness prime place among the commercially available means of body intervention. This goes beyond the body to involve the subject.

Just as the instrumentality of the fit body provides a marker of a better individual, more in control of herself, so, too, the 'naturalness' of being fit provides a marker of one's authenticity in willingly enduring fatigue for self-improvement. The effort required to improve the body makes it both more useful to the subject and also helps the subject avoid being 'unnatural'. This effort ensures that such transformations can be seen as legitimately acquired. Of course, even for fitness enthusiasts, absolute body plasticity – as promoted by the ever-growing increase of commercial body transformation techniques – seems to induce unease and curiosity at the same time. Fitness participants continually define the 'right' boundaries for body plasticity by drawing on what they have learnt in the gym about what fitness allows. Elena, a middle-aged clerical worker who trains regularly and with passion, sums it up well. 'It is not that I reject age or ageing, I think you must try to make the best of what you can'. She adds with conviction that 'external interventions' like plastic surgery, are not 'right'.

Voices like this seem to break away from the postmodern paradigm of absolute plasticity which sees women intent on transforming their bodies, solely concerned with pleasing others and indiscriminately greedy for everything which will serve that purpose (Bordo, 1993). Instead, the Italian gyms I investigated seem to express, perhaps, an older and modernist culture – certainly a less permissive and indulgent one. Women are not simply encouraged to choose the body they prefer, but to work diligently towards their own goals through disciplining themselves. Thus, for many of the women interviewed, especially the most enthusiastic and assiduous clients, learning to exercise signifies 'learning to give the utmost also in life', trying to 'improve oneself instead of complaining'. In other words, fitness is associated with personal liberation by applying traditionally bourgeois (and masculine) values including self-control and self-determination to the body, thereby demonstrating moral fibre. Despite a rhetoric which includes holistic concepts, such as 'well-being' and 'feeling good', fitness promotes that special form of body–self dualism typical of modern disciplinary techniques whereby better self-control is obtained not through mortification of the flesh, but by controlled stimulation of its capabilities.

In today's changing world, the body is often seen as the only area over which individuals may keep control or as the starting place to demonstrate one's superiority in times of hard social competition. Women's bodies have traditionally been considered (and disciplined) in their decorative features, men's in their functional qualities (West and Zimmerman, 1987). Now, decorative pressures on the female figure are shifting to assimilate functionality. For women no less than for men, an athletic, toned, docile body has become an important sign of virtue and character (Gillick, 1984; Glassner, 1992; Rader, 1991; White et al., 1995). The fit body has replaced the 1970s cult of thinness and the soft voluptuous curves of the early 1960s. The new composite ideal of the female body – strong and beautiful, muscular and slender, toned and shapely – contradicts the traditional association of femininity with immobility and passivity. Yet, while drawing women closer to the athletic image of an energetic and resolute subject, the main themes of fitness, namely body control and self-challenge, may also bring some women dangerously close to the obsessive worries of the anorectic and the compulsive exerciser, with all their attendant health risks (Yates, 1991).

Conclusion

Unlike the physical education rigidly organized by nation-states to govern their populace, contemporary commercial fitness culture now accessed by many groups of women responds to a mixed group of private subjects who want to enjoy themselves. They demand variety and novelty and can be persuaded but not coerced. This development may bolster the erroneous impression that caring for the body is something purely personal, not influenced by social organization, lacking in power implications and unleashed from rules. Yet, as this research illustrates, time training in the gym for these women is clearly not free from rules or from social consequences. Rather, it is well-organized productive time, producing physical changes and fostering a special notion of what is both natural and right to do for body and for self. If, as many clients claim, the time spent training is time for oneself, that self is not just *any* self. Fitness promotes a special vision of subjectivity, relatively independent of class and gender distinctions, but still linked to a moral image of self and the world. This image is characteristic of pluralistic and individualizing institutions which express modern culture, hinging on an idea of social mobility: with adequate work on oneself, anyone can obtain both a more disciplined body and social success.

In all the fitness activities studied, trainers prized effort, zeal and labour. They also stressed that the 'mere fact' of going to the gym 'with so many other things to do' is 'really a proof of value'. One client said that when she trains, she 'feels fit' and 'If I'm not more fit, at least I feel stronger and I feel better about myself'. Such a claim reinforces the idea that crucial to the fitness boom is women's opportunity to convey, both to themselves and to others, a satisfactory perception of a healthy self. While these preoccupations may be conducive to obsessive exercise behaviour, they also illustrate how far health goes beyond objective physical conditions, to reach into both personal and social ways of experiencing and portraying selves and bodies.

The idea of a fit body, useful to subjects in their daily lives and an immediate sign of self-control and adaptability, seems to have replaced previously modest fatalistic hopes of health (Sassatelli, 1999a and b). The very notion of health seems to have shifted from being defined as a fortuitous absence of disease to a set of capabilities which the subject can conquer (Crawford, 1985). This view attributes sole responsibility for care of the body to the individual, but underestimates everything that could possibly limit the efficacy of self-monitoring. In short, the subject comes to be seen as so strong that she may suddenly find herself unexpectedly carrying the whole weight of responsibility for her life, her physical defects and her ailments. Yet only such a strong subject, with full responsibility for her choices, will be seen as capable of choosing how to look after her body.

The framework of values discovered within keep-fit culture helps address some broader issues concerning women's health in contemporary Western societies. First, it shows that the notion of health cannot be taken for granted, since it is typically articulated in specific ways in different contexts. By closely examining the training setting and listening to the voices of participants, it was shown that, although fitness is increasingly portrayed as an healthy activity, it fosters only one particular view of health which is predicated on an instrumental notion of the body. Second, having appreciated how far the healthy form promised by fitness relates to morals, we can problematize the objectivity of the increasingly influential idea that health is something possible to be obtained by following self-imposed routines. This is particularly important for women. The female body has traditionally been seen not only as weak, but also as dangerous and risk-laden; it may now be seen as strong and safe – but only if women accept discipline themselves. Exercising the capacity to keep in good form is the price women must pay to be granted sovereignty over the body. Finally, the case of fitness culture illustrates that when women's health is discussed, what is at stake is not confined to technical notions of health. Having shown that the biomedical model is not morally and politically neutral (Turner, 1984), sociologists have often campaigned for wider views to be taken of health. However, it is not enough to adopt definitions which go beyond the absence of physical disease. These broader definitions are, themselves, clearly implicated in moral and political programmes of subjectivity and social order, which social scientists need also to address to engage effectively with women's health actions.

Further reading

Bordo, S., *Unbearable Weight. Feminism, Western Culture and the Body* (Berkeley: University of California Press, 1993).

Markula, P., 'Firm but Shapely, Fit but Sexy, Strong but Thin: The Postmodern Aerobicizing Female Bodies', *Sociology of Sport Journal*, 12 (4) (1995) 424–53.

Park, R.J., 'A Decade of the Body: Researching and Writing about The History of Health, Fitness, Exercise and Sport, 1983–1993', *Journal of Sport History*, 21 (1) (1994) 59–82.

Sassatelli, R., 'The Gym and the Local Organization of Experience', *Sociological Research Online* 4 (3) (1999) www.socresonline.org.uk/.

6
Listening Within: Counselling Women in Awareness of the Body

Judy Moore

Introduction

The promotion of women's well-being is increasingly recognized as a process in which women can actively determine rather than passively respond to contextual demands and dis-ease. Counselling is one way of supporting such a process. Over fifteen years working in the person-centred tradition of counselling, I have gradually learned that this form of counselling is less a psychological activity of unpicking the mind's constructions than creating an environment wherein the client is enabled to access the wisdom of her own body. In this chapter, I illustrate this process through the case study of a client whom I have called Bea. Her role as carer is one with which many women can identify and demonstrates how strong are the external pressures to conform to a role, rather than listen to the strong and subtle messages of our inner experiencing.

Counselling has become a recognized aspect of health care in developed countries in recent years, with many general practices in the United Kingdom now employing an accredited counsellor as part of their primary care team. The counsellor can help individuals who might otherwise be treated solely, and sometimes inappropriately, with medication, to explore the source of their depression or un-happiness to find their own way forward in difficult life-situations. Counselling can sometimes offer advantages over medication in dealing with serious life crises (McCormick, 1988) and, in some cases, over other traditional psychiatric interventions (Breggin, 1993). Counselling is increasingly offered in other health care contexts, most notably in the care of the terminally ill. Because of medical and public sector financial constraints, counselling is often time-limited, usually to six sessions, with strong pressure on counsellors to offer brief forms of therapy.

Most UK institutions of higher and further education now include counselling services in their student health and support provision, albeit with widespread present-day cuts, despite clear evidence of increasing distress and disturbance among the British student population (Rana et al., 1999). Fortunately our service was well resourced at the time I was seeing Bea, which enabled us to work at a much deeper level than an imposed time limit would have permitted.

The person-centred approach is just one of many counselling orientations to be found within primary health care settings and student welfare provision. Such practitioners may draw on cognitive, psychodynamic or systemic orientations and, increasingly, solution-focused brief therapy (Palmer, 2000). While the person-centred approach lends itself to both short- and long-term work, long-term work offers the greatest possibility for radical change and the nature of such change is my concern here.

Person-centred counselling involves the counsellor's offering to the client what are generally known as the 'core conditions' of the approach: congruence (being in touch with one's own flow of inner experiencing); empathy (the ability to track the client's flow of experiencing); and unconditional positive regard (a non-judgemental acceptance of all aspects of the client's experiencing). Where these conditions are experienced in the counselling relationship, constructive change in the client will occur. Misinterpretation of the core conditions has led to much misunderstanding of person-centred counselling. The apparent simplicity of the core conditions has led to them being often, and wrongly, regarded as skills that can be rapidly learned and superficially presented. Rather, I see them as embodying a way of being that offers a profound challenge to socially constructed views of right and wrong and of ways of living our lives according to those beliefs. To promote the habit of 'listening within' rather than listening to the prescriptive and judgemental voices that surround us, is the implicit task of the person-centred counsellor. At the same time, her explicit task is to enable the client to find her own way forward in terms of whatever situation has brought her to counselling.

The person-centred approach is predicated on a belief in the intrinsic goodness of human beings. The infant, unselfconsciously in touch with the flow of her inner experiencing, knows instinctively what she needs for her survival, but is dependent on others to meet those needs. As she grows up, she becomes increasingly aware of the views and expectations of the significant adults by whom her world is created, of other children and of the world encountered through the communications media. Where the positive regard of significant others is often conditional on her behaving in certain ways, she may become confused: her behaviour guided at times by wanting to please and at other times by the flow of inner experiencing. Carl Rogers, the founder of the person-centred approach (Thorne, 1992), discovered from extensive work in the field of child development at the outset of his career that the desire for positive regard would eventually prove stronger than the child's capacity to stay in touch with her inner experiencing. This is especially so in an environment where restrictive 'conditions of worth' are frequently imposed upon the child. As an adult, she is then likely to live her life according to the expectations and wishes of others.

It is often only through some life-crisis – a bereavement, a broken relationship, insurmountable difficulties at work – that the pain not only of the immediate crisis, but of living according to a false concept of self, may break through and, finally, bring her into counselling. Such pain and discomfort are manifestations of her inner life, the flow of experiencing with which she has almost lost touch. This is known in person-centred theory as the 'actualizing tendency', the directional flow within all beings that prompts us to move towards living in ways that are most life-enhancing and creative, to become most fully ourselves.

The process of person-centred therapy involves enabling the client to step back from what she may have become through her social environment to re-access her innate wisdom. Initially, Rogers formulated this inner wisdom specifically as *embodied* knowledge:

> 'You must let your experience tell you its own meaning' – when that sentence is deeply understood we will, in the writer's estimation, know much of what we wish to know in regard to psychotherapy. What is the usual alternative? It is to try to distort the many items of experience so that they fit in with the concepts... . we try to twist the sensations of vision, of hearing, of muscle tension, of heart beat, of gastric constriction to fit the partly true and partly false formulations which we have already built up in our consciousness. (Rogers, 1951: pp. 97–8)

This locates the most trustworthy knowing in an embodied, pre-verbal awareness that precedes the construction of our subjectivity through social discourse. Assimilating the basic meanings that arise in the body into the structure of self is made difficult within the distortions of our socially constructed world.

At the same time it is vital to be aware within the counselling process that women's lives and identity *are* profoundly and predictably shaped by the society in which we live. In relation to understanding 'the source of an individual's guilt, anxiety or depression', Walker writes:

> Recognizing both levels as significant, allows exploration of both internal and external worlds, acknowledging the power and respective influence of both. (Walker, 1990: p. 59)

While acknowledging the tension between inner experiencing and societal pressures, I here give more attention to aspects of inner experiencing. As a person-centred counsellor, I aimed simply to offer the core conditions, knowing that, in this particular therapeutic climate, Bea would eventually begin to access her own directional wisdom.

O'Hara has described Rogers and colleagues involved in formulating person-centred counselling as 'homeopathic psychologists' (Fairhurst, 1999: p. 64). Their approach is premised on a deep conviction that the client contains the resources for her own healing within herself, once she can accept the manifestations of her actualizing tendency. To listen to inner experiencing, in the face of cultural pressures to distract ourselves from this level of awareness, is a difficult task, and one which may feel personally risky. Nonetheless, undertaking it can ultimately challenge the social discourses that we have absorbed to hold ourselves in check, and bring about profound change (Moore and Hawtin, 1998).

It was not difficult for me to empathize and be fully accepting of Bea within the counselling relationship, but her process was much complicated and impeded by the series of crises and external pressures which confronted her at significant points just as she was beginning to experience internal change. It was particularly difficult to withstand the societal pressures on her to continue to 'cope' and to 'care' when she needed to turn her attention to herself.

The case study: Bea

I am grateful to Bea for her cooperation in the preparation of this study, which is based on notes made after every session and presents the essential details of her case, but with significant facts altered to preserve her anonymity.

I first met Bea three years ago when she sought counselling to help her deal with the pressures of caring for her mother, who had developed senile dementia. Bea, who is in her forties and a nurse by profession, was then in her second year at university and had recently moved into her mother's flat to care for her. She rented out her own house and lived in student accommodation for most of her first year until her mother's condition deteriorated so far that she could no longer take care of herself.

In the early sessions Bea talked about the isolation of her life with her mother. Although her mother attended day care five days a week and went away for occasional 'respite' weeks, Bea was her sole carer during evenings and weekends. Her mother veered from being the caring and affectionate person that Bea had always known to being suspicious that Bea was stealing from her and also being increasingly violent towards her. Bea would never know when her mother's next attack would come. Sometimes her mother would come into her bedroom at night and start hitting her when she was asleep. On one occasion, when her mother pulled Bea's hair, Bea hit her and felt extremely guilty about this.

Bea's brother (her only surviving close family member) was extremely unsupportive and, if Bea tried to tell him what was going on, he would respond by telling her to put her mother 'in a home'. At the same time, Bea's and her mother's friends and the medical professionals were all focused on her mother's welfare, ignoring what the process of caring might be doing to Bea herself. When Bea explained to her doctor that she was worried about the level of rage that she had begun to feel towards her mother during the outbursts of violence, he prescribed Prozac. This allopathic response was directly at odds with my commitment to working with Bea as a whole person and my belief that the way forward for her was to stay in touch with the truth of her experiencing. I was angry at the doctor's response, but was clear that it would have been inappropriate to share this response with Bea, in the desperate state she was then in. If she chose to accept the authority of the doctor at this point, that was what she needed to do and there was no doubt that her experience was indeed unbearable. Bea took the Prozac for several days, but stopped when she had a bad reaction to it, interestingly having already begun to develop her own self-protective mechanisms.

Bea talked about 'doubting [her] own sanity' as she tried to deal with her mother's accusations of stealing her money or her clothes and was aware of 'splitting off from [her] body' when her mother was hitting her. To survive, she was becoming increasingly removed from her own experiencing. My aim as her counsellor was to validate and enable her to return to that experiencing in all its complexity – an aim very much at odds with everyone else's aim, which seemed to be to keep her functioning at the most basic level as her mother's carer. Bea felt great relief at times as she contacted the depths of grief and rage that accompanied her sense of losing the mother she loved to a debilitating and frightening illness. At other times, she longed to shut out the pain and would herself collude in its denial by her friends and family. She would often arrive at counselling sessions saying she was 'fine', only gradually allowing herself to describe what had really been going on for her.

Over the weeks Bea began to contact a wider range of feelings and slowly, painfully, began to let go of the view, held by herself as well as others, that she was someone who could 'cope' with anything. Instead of breaking down into irrevocable chaos, as she had feared, she began to discover, even amidst the pain, a more vivid sense of being alive. By session 18, she had begun to 'enjoy little things' and to accept that it would be better for both of them if her mother went into residential care.

At this point, one of the long gaps, often a feature of counselling students, occurred. It is important to accept that the client, at such times, is likely to lose contact with the subtleties of her experiencing and to become more self-rejecting especially when she has been in an environment where she has not been heard. Bea missed several sessions because of bank holidays, exams and then a three-week trip with her mother to stay with Bea's brother in New Zealand. The holiday was a disaster from Bea's perspective, as her brother was distinctly unsupportive of her, becoming increasingly hostile towards both her mother and herself. On their return, Bea's mother's violence towards her increased and it was agreed, following a psychiatric assessment, that she should go into residential care.

The period following Bea's return was one of deepening despair. She began to believe that she was now 'beyond normality', incapable of relating properly to other people or leading a 'normal' life again. When an old friend came to stay she felt she had to put on a 'brave face' – a pattern that came to characterize her relating for the next two years. Bea's isolation intensified, even though she moved into a student house from her mother's flat and her emotional life found expression only in her counselling sessions where I tried to empathize with her despair and accept her need to fall back on old coping mechanisms.

As the pressures on her increased, with her mother's continuing deterioration in residential care and her final university year, Bea maintained her 'coping' façade. In residential care, her mother's violence was dealt with by increasing doses of medication, making her more dull and lifeless. What Bea had hoped was the best way forward for both of them had led to her mother losing the 'spark' which previously enabled her to enjoy some aspects of her life. Bea became increasingly despairing at her mother's situation. She was aware of curbing any longings for life to be anything more than joyless routine and I commented in my notes after one session: '[It's] as if her actualizing tendency has receded way back, surfacing only in grief and despair.'

Glimpses of anger about her mother's and her own situation eventually began to break through to become an overwhelming rage which Bea knew would be accepted without judgement in her counselling sessions, if not elsewhere in her life. Eventually, after several weeks, some sense of old longings and a more positive feeling for life began to stir. But, again, before Bea could stay for very long with these awakenings, the crisis with her mother deepened. Her condition rapidly deteriorated and she died at the Easter before Bea's final exams. Within weeks, the man Bea had once lived with for eight years also died and she was faced, through this double bereavement, with a sense of loss that seemed impossible to bear. The massive pressures of being her mother's carer were forgotten in her grief at losing the mother for whom she had tried so hard to do her best. She was angry at the treatment her mother had received at the end of her life and felt guilty for not having kept her at home.

At this critical point we met only infrequently, as Bea chose to focus her energies on getting through her exams. Meanwhile, her social isolation was deepening as she sought to push the feelings away. She talked about feeling 'as if in a cage', a cage that was 'so tightly locked [she] can never get out'. Although she talked about 'not needing' people, she longed for her mother and to be understood rather than to face platitudes about it being all 'being for the best'. Her own neediness was something she could only dimly perceive at this time during her very occasional counselling sessions.

Bea remained in her 'cage' for several months, working hard doing bank nursing and moving back into her own house. We did not begin to meet again regularly until the autumn when Bea returned to university to take another course. The process of uncovering her grief and pain began again, accompanied by a deep exhaustion that lasted for several months. Underneath all this was an anger so huge that it could not find adequate expression. In moving back to her old house, it was as if Bea had moved back into the life that she had left three years ago, when she first became a student and re-encountered the old frustrations that she had once sought to leave behind.

At university, Bea was perceived as a student, whilst among her family and old friends she was regarded as the person she used to be before the life-changing events of the previous three years. The truth of her experiencing as her mother's carer was invisible to all and could find no expression. Meanwhile her regular part-time work as a nurse was yet another version of being there for others with no apparent needs of her own. As her experiencing had become more complex, it had become ever more difficult to communicate, even to herself, and painstaking empathy was the only way forward. The next phase of our work in the counselling sessions was to access and process more of the events of the past three years and some of the old patterns that kept Bea fixed in her 'cage' even while raging at its constraints.

The difference now was that, however socially isolated she had become, Bea did value herself more, gradually becoming more aware of the strength of her negative feelings. She resented the invisibility that her role as 'carer' had brought upon her and was angry at what her time at university had become. Bea's fear of her own anger, now fuelled by so many different sources, directly related back to her fear of her father's anger. She had been greatly relieved when her parents divorced when she was twelve but the memory of her father's rages kept her own anger in check. She had no sense of how to begin to communicate anger without destroying herself or others. Her anger eventually erupted in fantasies about machine-gunning people down. She spoke about being 'tortured inside' by her bottled-up feelings. At times she expressed suicidal thoughts. But the depth of her despair remained invisible to everyone outside the counselling relationship.

The irony of Bea's situation was that she had been a 'carer' all her life – as a little girl, the placator of her father, a nurse for most of her adult life and finally her mother's principal carer through a rapid and frightening decline into dementia. Her determination to keep up a 'coping' façade was an old pattern brought to a situation with which no one else could cope. The fact that her mother was so soon sedated once in residential care is indicative of how extreme her condition had become and how impossible her daughter's task, while carrying on manifesting 'coping' behaviour. She was acting from a well-established self-concept at the expense of the truth of her own experiencing. The accumulation of caring roles pushed her ever further away from the wisdom of her body until being alive ceased to have meaning for her.

As she began to sense her feelings once again and to find them expression, the longing that had originally brought Bea to a new life at university began to reassert itself. Once she had allowed herself to experience within her body the extent of her overwhelming anger, despair and grief, she wanted it to be recognized by her family, friends and nursing colleagues. When her brother contacted her, she refused to deny her anger with him any longer and was clear that she would rather lose him than put up with anything for the sake of the relationship. She spoke more honestly to a colleague at work and then to two or three of her friends at the university. Each time she could be more open, she began to feel better. Each time she tried to speak and was misunderstood or her experiencing denied or belittled, she felt worse. Over the next few months, her feelings fluctuated violently but the intervals grew longer where she began to feel a little better and find a 'spark' of life beneath the painful feelings. It became evident to us both that she needed to be able to be more fully herself in a wider context than individual counselling sessions. Bea eventually joined a counselling group and began to spend more time with her university friends where the academic side of her personality could be received and she could finally begin to leave the 'carer' behind.

Bea was clearly beginning to outgrow her old life when she came to university, but the situation with her mother forced her back into one of her most deeply established patterns of behaviour. Like so many women, while longing to find herself, she had to be there for others and was conditioned to behave in ways appropriate to that role. I am confident that Bea has now begun to find a way forward and will live a fuller and richer life as a result of all that she has gone through. Had her situation been less painful or less extreme, she may not have been prompted to seek help and may never have worked beyond the roles to listen to who she really is.

Ignoring the wisdom of the body

What is evident from Bea's story is that cultural pressures, manifested most clearly in the reactions of her friends, family and the medical profession, converged to deny the truth of her own experiencing, of what she was feeling in her body.

Carl Rogers (1951) frequently compared personal growth to plant growth. As plants need certain conditions to grow and flourish, so do we, as human beings, need specific conditions (the 'core conditions') to become who we truly are. For the counsellor seeking to offer the core conditions, this means accepting all aspects of what is going on for the client, being empathically sensitive to what is expressed and also to what is at the *edge* of awareness – often a pre-verbal sensing – that may be harder to express. This is trying to 'tune in' to a level of experiencing that is generally unheard in Western culture, at which we nonetheless manifest our 'alive-ness'.

Only once Bea's anger had been accepted could she begin to experience the hurt that lay beneath the anger; on accepting that hurt she could begin to contact a deeper layer of grief; on accepting this grief, she could begin to sense another level of anger – and so on, until finally creating some space within all this pain should reawaken a sense of life that could begin to encompass hope and joy.

The denial of inner experiencing in the face of cultural conditioning and expectations could have condemned Bea to the mechanical living-out of her life, to suicide or to irremediably destructive patterns of relating to others. Her experience as a carer is particularly bad, but not uncommon in terms of the pressures and expectations often present in women's lives. Our response to these pressures depends on our own past and present social contexts. When our experiencing can be accepted and understood by those around us we can come through; when they deny or ignore our experiencing, we begin to doubt our own reality and may lose our sanity.

I suggest that the habit of diverting ourselves from what we are truly experiencing in our bodies is predominant in our culture, in daily pressures and even in conventions of everyday conversation. Once our experiencing feels incommunicable, the internal pressure is huge and the more deeply Bea became trapped in her 'cage' the more desperate she became. We cannot separate inner experiencing from external environment, but, as Walker points out, 'In today's society, the cult of the individual makes it all too easy to fall into the pit of self-blame' (1990: p. 59). As a counsellor, I need to recognize this cultural pattern while seeking to enable my clients to contact the as yet incommunicable edge of their experiencing which is deeper than the negativity of the 'pit' and beyond the entrapment of the 'cage'.

Accessing the wisdom of the body

The pressures to live according to convention and to subject ourselves to the distractions of an 'addictive society' (Schaef, 1989) can work powerfully against experiencing the body's messages. Learning to trust this level of experiencing is a difficult task which involves listening beneath layers of anger, hurt, guilt or self-blame which trap us further in the 'cage'. It also involves weighing up the relative risks entailed in staying in and attempting to leave the 'cage'.With his statement 'You must let your experience tell you its own meaning' Rogers makes it clear that he is talking about basic physiological sensations ('sensations of vision, of hearing, of muscle tension, of heart beat, of gastric constriction') to which we may attach 'feeling' labels that are either correct or incorrect (Rogers, 1951: pp. 97–8). If we could stay in tune with those sensations rather than denying them, we could live without 'inner strain' and move forward in a more positive and life-enhancing way for both ourselves and others. However, the 'addictive society' reduces the chances of our staying with the accuracy of inner experiencing so that, according to Rogers, basic needs 'become elaborated and channelized through cultural conditioning into needs which are only remotely based upon the underlying physiological tension' (Rogers, 1951: p. 492). Rogers' observations are even more applicable with today's ever greater array of distractions than at the time he wrote, and even though Rogers later began to talk about feelings in a much less precise way.

Within the counselling world, where talk of 'feelings' is commonplace, I find myself increasingly uncomfortable with the labelling of feelings as an end in itself. Through witnessing clients struggling to find an accurate word for what they are experiencing, I have become aware of how inadequate or misleading some of the 'feeling' labels can be. One 'feeling', once acknowledged, begins to shift into another (Bea's shifting from 'anger' to 'hurt' is an example of this). It is clear that, once this kind of movement has begun, the client is in a trustworthy process that will ultimately lead to her own healing.

A more refined description of inner process is provided in the writings of Gendlin, a colleague of Rogers in the 1950s, who has continued work on the significance of what goes on within us at a bodily level. He makes a careful distinction between a 'feeling' and what he calls the bodily 'felt sense' which is 'not a mental experience but a physical one'. This is 'not experienced as separate words or thoughts but as a single (though often puzzling and very complex) bodily feeling', therefore not 'easy to describe in words', and is 'an unfamiliar, deep-down level of awareness that psychotherapists (along with almost everybody else) have usually not found' (Gendlin, 1978/1981: pp. 32–3).

Gendlin explains that, through contacting this level of experiencing, we begin to expand into the fullness of who we are. It means acknowledging feelings, but also sensing beneath them and getting in touch with the flow of the actualizing tendency which is *in itself* deeply trustworthy. Gendlin's view is opposed to any social constructionist notion of the person. To adopt such a position, however, is very much at odds with our culture and the pressures and constraints it imposes, particularly upon those who hold least power in our society, more often including women. Within a role such as that of carer, women are subject to definitions absorbed with our cultural heritage and, without consistent validation, we can lose sight of who we are beneath that role.

Conclusion

When counselling women, I know that I need to be aware of the extreme tension that exists between inner experiencing and the external pressures that construct a significant part of our identity. My task as a counsellor is to validate a level of experiencing that is generally left unheard and to acknowledge that it may sit at odds with what other people hear and see. This begins a process that is irreversible, however lost it may become at times. In terms of person-centred personality theory, it means living from the actualizing tendency rather than the self-concept or, in more general terms, living from the *truth* of who we are rather than *what we have been told we are.* To begin to live in this way reclaims our bodies as the repository of our deepest wisdom and offers women the most profound challenge to our present culture that we can make.

Further reading

Gendlin, E., *Focusing*, revised edn. (New York: Bantam Books, 1978/1981)
Gendlin, E., *Focusing-Oriented Psychotherapy: A Manual of the Experiential Method* (New York: Guilford Press, 1996).
Rogers, C., *Client-Centered Therapy* (London: Constable, 1951).
Thorne, B., *Carl Rogers* (London: Sage,1992) (pp. 24–43 for the best brief account of Rogerian theory).

Part III

Giving Women a Voice: The Power of Health Dialogues

7
Professional Control or Women's Choice in Childbirth? Is Either Possible?

Wendy Savage

Introduction

Over the last 50 years, the relationship between doctors and patients has changed dramatically. The paternalistic approach, seeing the patient as a passive recipient of the care prescribed by the doctor, who 'knew best', has changed as the autonomy of patients has come to be seen as an important factor in their care. They are acknowledged as having a right to be kept fully informed about the options for care and to take part in shared decision-making (General Medical Council, 1995). How this can be achieved in women's reproductive health is a matter for debate, as midwifery has become more dominated by obstetricians since, at the time of writing, home birth has become uncommon. The majority of obstetricians and gynaecologists are men and so have only theoretical, second-hand, not experiential, knowledge of women's health problems. Their focus on mortality and technology, rather than the psychological and emotional aspects of childbirth, may be seen to reflect a more masculine approach to life.

Childbirth is not an illness. Nevertheless, women may die as a result and continue to do so in large numbers in the developing world. Doctors, therefore, do have a role to play in the improvements in both maternal and perinatal mortality over the last 50 years. These improvements are seen by most doctors as resulting from the transfer of childbirth from the home under the care of midwives and family physicians, to hospital care directed by obstetricians. The dissatisfaction of women in the United Kingdom with the lack of alternatives to this approach was finally heard in 1991 by a Parliamentary Select Committee (House of Commons Health Committee, 1992). The UK government's response to its report, *Changing Childbirth* (Department of Health, 1993), recommended that women should have more choice and control over childbirth. The result of this policy change has been a modest increase in home births from 1 per cent to 2 per cent and an increasing rate of Caesarean section (CS), which is said to be due to women exercising choice over the mode of delivery (Jackson and Irvine, 1998). The issue of home birth provides one example of the exercise of professional control, as does the debate over whether it is women or obstetricians who are choosing CS rather than vaginal delivery.

Important questions raised by these changes are: what the role of a professional may be; how far obstetricians have relinquished control over childbirth; whether choice without responsibility is possible; and whether professional control can coexist with women's choice in childbirth. In addressing these questions, this chapter draws on studies and reports from the UK and US to exemplify the issues of the organization of maternity services, the place of birth, and the rising rate of CS. It also reflects the author's 35 years' experience as a practising obstetrician and gynaecologist in London, Nigeria, Kenya and New Zealand, visits to China, Russia, Yugoslavia, Hungary, and having a baby in the US in 1964 (Savage, 1986).

Recent history of maternity services in the UK

The Parliamentary Select Committee mentioned above, chaired by Nicholas Winterton, published a seminal report about maternity services in 1992. For the first time, a UK government committee had not only listened to, but also accepted, the views of women who use maternity services. Over the previous 30 years, a revolution in maternity care had quietly deprived women of the choice about where to have their babies and of control over the way their babies were born. Yet this was at a time when the involvement of people in decisions about their own medical care generally was becoming far more acceptable to society and the professions (General Medical Council, 1993). The Winterton Committee stated that there was no evidence that having a baby in hospital was safer than having it at home. It pointed to the expressed preferences of women for choice, continuity and proper communication. It commented on how the three professional groups looking after women, GPs, midwives and consultant obstetricians, appeared to be in conflict, losing sight of the woman's needs, which should be the focus of care. The evidence given by the Association for the Improvements of Maternity Services (AIMS) and the National Childbirth Trust was well researched and evidence-based; women talked movingly of their unsympathetic treatment by doctors. In contrast, the submission of the Royal College of Obstetricians and Gynaecologists (RCOG), based on opinion rather than evidence, was not well received by the Committee (Declercq, 1998).

The medical and social models of childbirth

Radical change in maternity care in the 1960s had been based on the assumption by obstetricians that the medical model, in which they had been trained to be the experts, was applicable to all women, whether healthy or sick. This model supports the view that no pregnancy is normal, except in retrospect. The alternative, a social model, recognizes the fundamental social and psychological significance of birth as an event embedded in society, an intimate part of the woman's and her family's lives. Here, pregnancy is seen as a normal physiological event, unless something goes wrong.

Maternal and perinatal mortality: the safety of childbirth

Childbirth in the UK has never been safer. Figure 7.1 shows the rates of maternal mortality in England and Wales from 1850 to 1970.

Since 1980, the rate has largely remained at about 8 per 100,000, recently rising to 12 per 100,000, probably due to better ascertainment of cases (Department of Health et al., 1998). This equates to the risk of dying in a road accident. In contrast, from the 1800s to 1935–40 the rate had varied between 4 to 6 per 1,000 (Loudon, 2000). So, when I was born, my mother's chance of dying in childbirth was about 1 in 250. In the developing world, the lifetime risk of dying in association with childbirth may be as high as 1 in 25 (World Health Organization, 1989). One can see that whilst women were and are dying at such a high rate, the professionals have concentrated on the business of preventing unnecessary maternal deaths. Obstetricians contributed to the fall in the UK, with their triennial Confidential Enquiries into Maternal Deaths, started in the 1950s (DHSS, 1989). Once they had reduced maternal mortality, by the 1970s, the attention of UK doctors moved to the baby.

The perinatal mortality rates (PMR) in England and Wales, the North East Thames and all women (not just our booked patients) at the London Hospital, from 1975 to 1991, are shown in Figure 7.2. The perinatal mortality rate is defined as the number of stillbirths and deaths in the first week of life per 1,000 total births. This figure

Figure 7.1   Maternal mortality in England and Wales from 1850–1980

Year	Maternal Mortality Rate
1850	5.5
1855	4.7
1860	4.7
1865	5
1870	4.8
1875	5.4
1880	6
1890	4
1885	4.8
1890	4.7
1895	4.6
1900	4.7
1905	4.3
1910	3.5
1915	4.1
1920	4.3
1925	4
1930	4.4
1935	4.6
1940	4
1945	2.5
1950	1.7
1955	1.1
1960	0.5
1965	0.3
1970	0.2

Source: Figures from Loudon (2000).

covers the rate until 1991, when the definition of stillbirths changed from 'births under 28 weeks' (from the last menstrual period) to 'births under 24 weeks', when very premature babies are less likely to survive, sending up the rate and losing continuity. In 1975, about

Figure 7.2   Perinatal mortality rate in England and Wales, North East Thames Region and the London Hospital (all women, not just booked patients)

Year	England and Wales	North East Thames Region	The London Hospital
1975	19.2	19.3	17.8
1976	17.5	18.7	17.8
1977	17	17.6	16.6
1978	15.5	15	21.3
1979	14.7	12.5	26.3
1980	13.3	13.1	23.6
1981	11.7	10.7	16.4
1982	11.3	11.4	14.6
1983	10.4	9.3	15.6
1984	10.1	8.9	14.1
1985	9.8	8.8	9.5
1986	9.5	9.5	10.2
1987	8.9	8.6	10.2
1988	8.7	9.1	11.9
1989	8.3	8.2	7.5
1990	8.1	8.5	7.3
1991	8	8.2	8.1
1992	7.9	7.1	9.3
1993	8.9	9.7	14.5
1994	8.9	9.5	14
1995	8.8	9.1	9.8
1996	8.6	9	9.6

Source: Figures from 1995 OPCS Childhood, Perinatal and Infant Mortality Statistics and London Hospital Obstetric database.

20 babies per 1,000 were dying in association with birth; by 1991, this was down to just under 10. Women in Britain today have a better chance of emerging from pregnancy safely and with a live baby than ever before (Department of Health et al., 1998; Office for National Statistics, 1998).

Women's increasing dissatisfaction with maternity care

The place of birth

Births moved from home to hospital in the 1960s. Whereas in 1958 over a third of women had their babies at home, by 1980 this was true for only 1 per cent. As the medical model of childbirth took over, midwives lost their traditional role. The work of sociologists in the 1960s and 1970s helped voice women's dissatisfaction about, for example, the large number of people seen during antenatal care, 'cattle market' antenatal clinics, and impersonal hospital services (Graham et al., 1999; McIntyre, 1976; Oakley, 1984; Roberts, 1981).

Campbell et al. (1983) analysed home births in England and Wales in 1979 when the Perinatal Mortality Rate (PMR) was 14.9 per 1,000. For booked home births, the PMR was low, at about 4 per 1,000. Those women who had booked at hospital but delivered unexpectedly at home had a PMR of 67.5 per 1,000, and the women who had not booked had a PMR of 196.6. As ever fewer women planned to have their babies at home, their good results were outweighed by the unplanned home births. The only Western country which has contin-ued a tradition of births at home (37 per cent) is the Netherlands, where the overall PMR is much the same as the UK and where the results of their midwives have been excellent (Treffers et al., 1990).

Government advice about the place of birth

In 1959, the Cranbrook Committee, in which medical advisers out-numbered civil servants, recommended that domiciliary midwifery should be maintained, but that 70 per cent of births should be enabled to take place in hospital (Ministry of Health, 1959). In the 1950s, a postwar bulge of births and a consequent lack of maternity beds had forced a number of women to have their babies at home. By 1970, the government had achieved its objectives, with 67.6 per cent of births taking place in hospital, 18.5 per cent in GP units and only 12.3 per cent at home. The Peel Committee (Short Report, 1980) made a classic epidemiological mistake about home births, stating that it was now safer to have a baby in hospital forgetting that half the home deliveries were unintended and had a high PMR.

The policy of the Royal College of Obstetricians and Gynaecologists was also that home was a dangerous place and everybody should have their babies in hospital. Between 1969 and 1989, the proportion of deliveries supervised by GP obstetricians fell from almost 30 per cent to about 4 per cent. It is interesting that published statistics never provided information on midwives, yet midwives were the senior people at the delivery in about 80 per cent of all births. By 1980, only one woman in 200 was having a planned home birth and many women who said they wanted to have their baby at home reported that their family practitioners (GPs) had struck them off their lists (Lloyd's evidence, House of Commons Health Committee, 1992, p. 912). If such women lived in a rural area with no alternative GP within easy distance, this would have posed problems. However, UK midwives do have a statutory duty to attend a woman in childbirth, even if she decides to have her baby at home against their advice, or that of the obstetrician or GP.

The Cumberledge Committee, 1993; a changing climate

The government responded to the Winterton Committee's report by setting up an expert maternity group chaired by Julia Cumberledge. Its report, *Changing Childbirth*, had many recommendations, including that: midwives should be the lead professional for a third of women and should have beds in the hospital; all women should hold their own medical notes; 75 per cent of women should be delivered by somebody whom they know; and no midwifery team should be larger than six members (Department of Health, 1993). Although these 'indicators of success' were due to be reviewed after five years (in 1998), this has not yet happened. In the meantime, the Royal College of Obstetricians and Gynaecologists, while not retreating far from their position that hospital birth is safer (Drife, 1999; RCOG, 1992), have, none the less, made a point of incorporating user views to the effect that home birth is an acceptable option for which appropriate information should be provided (RCOG, 1993). As a result of this changing climate, midwives generally appear to feel more self-confident, and many women do feel more in control. Control has been found to be very important in women's satisfaction with the outcome of pregnancy (Green et al., 1988).

The 1994 Home Birth Study

Following the Cumberledge Report, a major survey carried out in 1994 matched a cohort of 6,044 women at 37 weeks' pregnancy, who were planning home births, with a group of similar age and parity, who had decided on hospital birth (Chamberlain et al., 1996). Slightly more of the women planning to have their babies at home were of a higher social class. This, the most recent study, shows that home birth was safe for both mother and baby, and that intervention rates such as

Caesarean section and assisted vaginal deliveries were halved in those booked for home birth. Analysis of a sample of women completing a questionnaire at six weeks, showed that almost 95 per cent of the women who had home births managed to breast feed initially, with 65 per cent continuing to do so at the follow-up. This was almost twice the rate for the women who had their babies in hospital. That may be to do with the women's choice, but it may also be related to how the women felt about the whole birth process, and how encouragement by a midwife they knew enhanced the process and their confidence. A further area where women now appear to be exercising choice is that of operative delivery (Jackson and Irvine, 1998; Wilkinson et al., 1998; Graham et al., 1999; MacKenzie, 1999).

Caesarean section

The recent increase in the rate of Caesarean sections has been seen by some obstetricians as a result of women exercising their choice in childbirth and being encouraged to have a planned operative delivery (Paterson-Brown and Fisk, 1999). This is a prime example of an issue which raises questions about informed choice and the way in which women may be presented with the options.

The rise in the Caesarean section rate

Figure 7.3 shows the Caesarean section rate (CSR) in three countries – England and Wales (E and W), the US and Holland – since the 1970s.

Figure 7.3 Caesarean section rate in three countries: USA, England and Wales, and the Netherlands, 1970–92

Year	1970	1975	1980	1985	1990	1992
USA	5.5	10.4	16.5	22.7	23.8	23.4
England and Wales	4.9	6	9.5	10.5	12.1	13.1
Netherlands	2.1	2.7	4.7	5.7	6.7	7.8

Source: Constructed from: Clark and Taffel (1996: 166–8) (USA); Appendix of Winterton Report (England and Wales); Treffers, Eskes, Kleiverda and van Alten (1990: 2203–8) (the Netherlands)

In 1970, there was little difference between the US and England and Wales, but by 1990, the US rate was more than twice that of England and Wales. That was entirely due to the different practice in the US: 'once a Caesar always a Caesar' was the rule for subsequent childbirth management, whereas in the UK women were allowed to try for a vaginal delivery after one Caesarean operation. The US public health physicians became anxious in the late 1970s when the rate had tripled, and set up a task force to look at it (Task Force, 1981). Although this recommended that vaginal birth after CS should be allowed, it took several years to become accepted policy in the United States. By 1990, the US government had issued targets for the reduction of the CS rate and for raising the proportion of women attempting vaginal birth after CS (Department of Health and Human Services, 1991).

Breech presentation: an example of professional control or women's choice?

Because obstetricians in the UK always accepted a trial of vaginal delivery after one CS, the rate did not increase as rapidly as in the US. Since the publication of *Changing Childbirth* in 1993, some obstetricians have asserted that CS has been the choice of many women. However, what information is given to the woman, and how it is given, are crucial. For example, a woman with a breech presentation, told that there is a higher perinatal mortality and morbidity, that the baby is going to die or the head may get stuck, may find it much harder to persist with a choice of vaginal delivery (Waites, 1999).

Although the MIDIRS Informed Choice leaflet on breech delivery (Midwives Information and Resource Service with the University of York Centre for Reviews and Dissemination, 1997) leaves the choice of delivery route to the woman, evidence is not provided to support the woman's choice of CS. There is evidence that vaginal breech delivery in experienced hands is a safe option for mother and baby (Irion et al., 1998) and that it is safer for the mother to have a vaginal delivery than a CS (Lilford, 1990). There is, at present, a randomized controlled trial recruiting women to provide definitive evidence for outcomes of the vaginal breech as compared with elective CS (Hannah and Hannah, 1996). Breech delivery exemplifies the problems for lay women of reading and interpreting a voluminous literature from which professionals may reach completely different views.

Women should know that their chance of having a CS for a breech presentation may be doubled according to the policy of their consultant obstetrician. In my hospital, rates for women with breech presentations who deliver successfully vaginally, are: two-thirds of those booked under me; half of those booked under the colleague with whom I work most closely; and a third of those booked under my other colleagues. However, when the London Hospital midwives in 1997 suggested that we consultants might send a statement to the family physicians about obstetricians' policies, everybody, apart from myself, opposed this.

Such clinical decision-making is still kept behind closed doors and under professional control. Few hospitals report their rates of intervention.

Obstetricians' views about the rising Caesarean section rate

Colin Francome and I questioned obstetricians in 1990 (Savage and Francome, 1993) about why they thought that the CS rate had risen, following Francome's earlier study (Francome, 1989). The most commonly given reason was the better survival of premature babies, making CS a worthwhile option for a different group of women. However, as only about 1.8 per cent of women actually have their babies at 32 weeks or below, where neonatal intensive care has made such a difference, this would not explain the almost doubled rate of the 1970s. McIwaine (1985) showed that, at that time, CS for very premature babies made up only 2 per cent of all the Caesarean sections in Scotland, where the rate varied between hospitals from 5 to 19 per cent. She concluded that the differences were mainly due to the attitude of the obstetricians.

'Reduction in difficult forceps delivery' had been mentioned by 13 per cent in Francome's earlier study, but was hardly mentioned by 1990. 'Repeat Caesareans' accounted for 12 per cent of reasons in 1983, yet by 1990 this had fallen to 3 per cent, while the number of primary Caesareans had increased. Most shocking was that, whereas in 1983 litigation was the third most commonly given reason at 28 per cent, by 1990 it was the major reason given for the rise in CS. A woman being advised to have a CS would not have this explained to her by the obstetrician. As a former Director of Maternal and Child Health in the WHO European region says, 'It is an obscene thought that the doctor is going to pull the baby out or cut your baby out because he is frightened of being sued' (personal communication, but issues discussed in Wagner, 1994). Surely this is not what being a professional is all about.

Giving information

How can we explain risk to women and share uncertainty? This is essential if we are to be honest with them and help them understand what is going on in labour. However, simply saying to a woman that her baby is in danger is likely to ensure she will agree to almost anything. Thornton and Lilford (1989) showed that when informed of a risk of 1 in 20,000 to the baby, women would opt for a CS. Yet this risk is higher following a CS, at about 1 in 5,000 (Hall, 1994, p. 91). A professional has a duty of care, both to the woman and her baby, and a role to exercise objective judgement at a time when her judgement may be distorted owing to pain or sedation.

For doctors, performing a CS is an easier option than dealing with the uncertainty of a labour that is not straightforward. Particularly in these days of fragmented training, they may not see the woman after surgery, nor the difficulties the woman may have coping with the baby after a major operation with a scar on the abdomen.

Obstetricians have now begun to report that women are requesting elective CS because of fear of damage to the pelvic floor, following media interest in a small study published as a letter in the *Lancet* (Al-Mufti et al., 1996). A minority appears to be fuelling these fears (personal communications from RCOG members). However, an editorial in the *British Journal of Obstetricians and Gynaecology* concluded that choosing CS to protect the pelvic floor could not be justified (Sultan and Stanton, 1996). By 1999, the Ethics Committee of the International Federation of Gynaecology and Obstetrics (FIGO, 1999) was so concerned at the trend towards choosing CS for non-medical reasons that it issued a statement concluding that this practice could not be justified ethically because of a lack of good data, the risks of surgery, the after-effects and the extra cost. They concluded that normal vaginal delivery is safer in the short and long term for mother and child.

Conclusion

The role of a professional is to keep up to date with the knowledge and research in the field, to communicate effectively, to maintain the necessary skills and to acknowledge where information is lacking – in other words, to admit uncertainty. The advice that professionals give should be based on evidence and be in the best interests of the patient. It does not seem that obstetricians have substantially relinquished control over childbirth, although their power may have been somewhat reduced in the UK by managerial changes. They still largely control the organization of maternity services, even if midwives are more influential than formerly. Women in the UK have little choice about how services are provided despite government rhetoric, for example, about Patients' Charters (Department of Health, 1992). The option of home birth is still denied to many women who would prefer it. 'Domino' schemes, where women are visited and assessed at home by the midwife, transferred to hospital for the birth and return home after six hours, have been unable to run in recent years because of the shortage of midwives.

A woman's freedom to choose also brings responsibility. However, such responsibility requires full, not over-selective or persuasive information, so that she can make an informed choice (Kirkham, 1999). The Informed Choice leaflet produced by the Midwives Information and Resource Service (MIDIRS) and the Centre for Research and Dissemination at York are an excellent start. One, which contains all the recent references to evidence, is provided for the professional. There is another for the woman, which omits the references, is in simpler language, but gives access to the professional's leaflet if she wishes it (MIDIRS, 1997). If a woman with a complicated pregnancy decides to deliver at home, despite clear advice from her doctor and midwife of the potential problems in doing this, she must take responsibility if the outcome is not good. Deciding to complain about the professionals, or to sue them with the benefit of hindsight, is rare, but abrogates parental responsibility.

The title of this chapter posed the question, 'Professional control or woman's choice: is either possible?' The answer is not quite as simple as this polemical question would suggest. What we need is mutual respect and trust so that there is cooperation and not confrontation between the various people involved in maternity care. There have been changes in the obstetric profession. My experience of doctors in training suggests they are now much more willing to listen to women's views, and to let their wishes, if not taking precedence, at least be considered in their advice.

However, a continuing threat to both professionals and women in the UK is the issue of the management of the health services. Many small maternity units, whose flexibility is often preferred by women, have been closed by health authorities on economic grounds over the last 20 years. Good pilot schemes of teams of caseload midwifery care have not been continued despite their success. The Edgware Birth Centre faces an uncertain future, despite its popularity. A widespread shortage of midwives has led to women being denied preferred hospital places or home births. The pressure to discharge women from hospital, with little time to see how they have coped with the pregnancy and birth, is a real threat to both the professionals and the women. The majority of women do not demand to have a certain type of care, but do want to be able to reach an informed opinion of what will be best for themselves and their babies, with the best advice from the professionals they meet.

In conclusion, although the medical profession, like society in general, has been male-dominated, affecting the way services have been organized, relationships between doctors and patients are changing from a paternalistic to a more equal relationship. Choice is now on the agenda. But the spotlight must now turn to the issues of informed choice and to the limits of choice in an increasingly consumerist world. Will the health professions survive – or will women with internet printouts come to view the professionals merely as childbirth technicians?

Further reading

Kitzinger, S., *Re-discovering Birth* (Boston; New York; London: Little Brown, 2000).

Francome, C., Savage, Churchill W.H. and Lewison, H., *Caesarean Birth in Britain – A Book for Health Professionals and Parents* (Middlesex University Press in association with The National Childbirth Trust, 1993).

Tew, M., *Safer Childbirth? A Critical History of Maternity Care* (London; New York; Tokyo; Melbourne; Madras: Chapman and Hall, 1990).

Wagner, M., *Pursuing the Birth Machine* (Camperdown, NSW, Australia: Ace Graphics, 1994).

8
Pregnant Women and Consent to Treatment – From Autonomy to State Control and Back Again

Barbara Hewson

> Fetal rights cases – from forced medical treatment to drug abuse cases – represent attempts by the state to assert its control over women's bodies.
>
> (Daniels, 1993: p. 138)

Women's choices during pregnancy can arouse controversy. My concern is the way in which the law has been used as an instrument for restricting pregnant women's choices, on the ground that their conduct imperils their foetuses. While the law is generally (or appears to be) gender-neutral, it has been deployed in a manner that is not gender-neutral. At a time when women in Western democracies are enjoying greater social, legal and economic freedom than ever before, legal processes have been invoked to detain, punish or even assault pregnant women. Courts have been asked to detain pregnant women whose mental health problems or drug addictions are seen as a threat to the foetus; to punish women who have taken alcohol or other drugs during pregnancy; or to compel pregnant women who refuse obstetric intervention to undergo forced medical treatment. A number of such cases succeeded, particularly in the United States. This chapter will concentrate on developments in English courts, with some reference to American cases.

These cases raise troubling questions about women's autonomy: Does a woman forfeit her autonomy because she is pregnant; and if so, what is the justification? An assumption underlying these cases is that a pregnant woman is an inferior being, whose fundamental rights to bodily integrity and liberty can be infringed in pursuit of a 'higher' good, namely, the well-being of her foetus. I would argue that such an assumption reflects what some would like the law to be rather than the

116

law as it is. In classic theories of liberty, the guiding principle is that people should be free to do as they please, provided that they do not harm others. It is also a guiding principle of English law that people are free to do what they like, provided that it is not illegal. Typically, our laws do not explicitly regulate pregnant women's conduct by reference to the foetus. Nor does the law recognize the foetus as a legal person. Thus, a pregnant woman is free to drink, smoke, take drugs and undergo or refuse medical treatment as she pleases. Even if such conduct elicits moral disapproval, she is free to be 'bad'. The only express prohibitions which pregnant women face are laws criminalizing abortion or induced miscarriage. In most Western countries, such laws have been modified to permit abortions on medical or social grounds.

Cases in which the law is used to coerce, and sometimes punish, pregnant women are linked with a backlash against abortion, and abortion rights, prevalent in the US. A tenet of the anti-abortion movement is that pregnant women must sacrifice their autonomy in the service of their foetuses. One of its strategies is to use legal processes to give foetuses a more elevated moral and legal status. Anti-abortion supporters argue that foetuses are children, who merit full legal 'personhood'. This succeeded in South Carolina, in 1997, when the Supreme Court there declared that a viable foetus is a legal person (Paltrow, 1999: 1029–35). Whitner was imprisoned for eight years for child neglect as a result of taking cocaine during pregnancy (*Whitner* v *State*, 1997). She appealed. The Supreme Court dismissed her appeal, concluding that child neglect laws include foetuses. South Carolina's Attorney General then stated: '*Whitner* must now be construed as part of South Carolina's abortion statutes.' His office argued that post-viability abortions could be prosecuted as murder, and those involved receive the death penalty (Paltrow, 1999: pp. 1005, 1035).

Whitner remains exceptional, and it is highly unlikely that it would be followed in the United Kingdom. Overall, the law does respect women's autonomy, but only if women are given a proper opportunity to argue their cases, in the same way as other litigants. The law has proved susceptible to manipulation by state authorities, which often overlook legal precedent when seeking to coerce pregnant women, frequently in rushed hearings in which women are either absent, or unable to present their case effectively. I shall briefly explain the US legal scene first, because US cases have been used in attempts to curb pregnant women's autonomy in English courts. The US cases form part of the reaction to the US Supreme Court's famous decision in *Roe* v *Wade* (1973) and later abortion rulings. The US abortion cases are complex. Put simply, they acknowledge that a pregnant woman has a constitutionally protected right to terminate her pregnancy. The US Supreme Court also decided that the state is entitled to restrict women's access to abortion, at foetal viability. It did not accept that viable foetuses are 'persons', however. The Supreme Court said instead that, once a foetus is viable, the state acquires a compelling interest in protecting foetal life. But even when a foetus is viable, the Supreme Court has held that a woman must be permitted access to an abortion if this is necessary to protect her life or health. At this point, the state is not permitted to 'trade off' the woman's interests in preserving her life or health, against the continued survival of the foetus (*Thornburgh* v *American College of Gynecologists*, 1986; *Planned Parenthood* v *Casey*, 1992).

Foetal rights theorists put a novel spin on this reasoning. They argue that, if the state can restrict late abortion to cases where the woman's health or life requires it, the state is also entitled to take invasive measures to protect viable foetuses. Some theorists also argue that a woman should ensure the mental and physical health of her child at birth, on pain of civil or even criminal liabilities. Janet Gallagher, an American feminist lawyer, reviewed the extensive literature in this field (Gallagher, 1987). She argues that foetal rights theories represent a serious distortion of the *Roe* v *Wade* doctrine. She regards *Roe* v *Wade* as a powerful constitutional affirmation of individual autonomy (Gallagher, 1987: p. 15). She also warns that, for foetal rights theorists, foetal viability is not the endpoint for state interference in pregnant women's lives. They want the state to 'appropriate the woman's body and life to the affirmative service of the fetus', from conception onwards (Gallagher, 1987: pp. 42–3).

In the US, foetal rights theories were used as a basis for attacking women's civil liberties in various court actions. Some cases involved forced obstetric intervention; or lawsuits against women who allegedly harmed their foetuses *in utero* (for example, by taking medicine, or having sexual intercourse); or prosecutions of pregnant women addicted to drugs or alcohol for allegedly inflicting foetal harm. Often, the women involved were poor, black or Hispanic (see Gallagher, 1987; Kolder et al., 1987). Court hearings were sometimes rushed, with the women having little or no chance to articulate their constitutional rights effectively. Cases of forced obstetric intervention ceased in 1990, following a multi-million dollar lawsuit by the estate of Angela Carder. Angela was a pregnant cancer sufferer, who died after judges forced non-consensual Caesarean surgery on her (*Re AC*, 1987). Angela was prepared to consider surgery when her foetus was more mature. The judges knew that surgery would shorten her life, but they reasoned that she was going to die anyway. There was a slim chance that the 26-week old foetus would survive premature Caesarean delivery, but it did not. Angela's appeal was heard posthumously. In a landmark ruling, the District of Columbia Court of Appeals ruled that a pregnant woman was free to refuse medical treatment, even if she were near death and even if a refusal would jeopardize her foetus (*Re AC*, 1990). It noted that previous decisions ordering forced obstetric intervention had failed to address the critical question of pregnant women's constitutional rights. Two Illinois courts later ruled that forced treatment of pregnant women was unlawful (*Re Doe*, 1994; *Fetus Brown*, 1997). These decisions reinforce Gallagher's point that, when arguments for forced intervention are thoroughly tested against constitutional standards, they do not pass muster.

More recently, an estimated 200 women addicted to drugs while pregnant have been arrested in over 30 US states, on theories of foetal abuse (NARAL, 2001; Paltrow, 1999). Child abuse laws were given strained interpretations to include foetuses within the word 'child'. The women were frequently also victims of racial and social prejudice. Sentencing one woman in 1994, a South Carolina judge said that he was 'sick and tired of these girls having these *bastard* babies on crack cocaine' (Paltrow 1999: 1051). Judge Eppes said: 'we've got enough trouble with normal children. Now this little baby's born with crack. When he is seven years old, they have an attention span that long. [Holding his thumb and index finger an inch apart]. They can't run. They just run around in class like a little rat. Not just black ones. White ones too' (Paltrow, 1999: pp. 1025–6). In South Carolina and California, addicted pregnant women attending ante-natal clinics have been arrested and prosecuted rather than offered treatment. In 2001, the US Supreme Court allowed an appeal by ten women arrested while seeking maternity care at the MUSC hospital in Charleston, South Carolina. The women were covertly tested for drugs and tested positive for cocaine (*Ferguson* v *City of Charleston*, 2001); they were reported to the police, and arrested. All but one of the 30 women were African-American. One was kept shackled for two days during labour and delivery. Others were arrested after giving birth and removed to prison. The US Supreme Court ruled that testing pregnant women for law enforcement purposes, without their consent and without a warrant, was unconstitutional.

In the *Whitner* case mentioned earlier, Whitner, an African-American, was convicted of criminal child neglect for allegedly failing to provide proper medical care for her unborn child. He was born healthy, but a test indicated pre-natal exposure to cocaine. There were no in-patient residential drug programmes for pregnant drug users when she was charged in 1992. She had a court-appointed trial attorney, who met her on the day of her trial. She pleaded guilty and was sentenced to eight years in prison. No treatment was offered to her. Her appeal initially succeeded, but in 1997 a majority of the South Carolina Supreme Court declared that a viable foetus is a 'person' covered by child abuse laws. The majority accepted that, as a result of their ruling, such laws could be used to punish pregnant women who drank or smoked. The majority's decision was heavily criticized by two dissenting judges, one of whom was the Chief Justice. His co-dissenter complained: 'the impact of today's decision is to render a pregnant woman potentially criminally liable for myriad acts which the legislature has not seen fit to criminalize' (*Whitner*, 788). Thus, being overweight, failing to take exercise, taking too much exercise or drinking coffee could all potentially expose pregnant women to criminal sanctions. In Wisconsin, judges rejected the argument that a pregnant woman could be taken into protective custody for the sake of her foetus (*State of Wisconsin ex rel. Angela MW*, 1997). The Wisconsin legislature retaliated by passing a law which permits the authorities to detain a woman suspected of harming her foetus by 'habitual lack of self control in the use' of alcohol, and other drugs.

In the UK, the legal experience has been much less dramatic. There have no comparable attempts to criminalize women for their conduct while pregnant. There has been only one reported attempt to detain a pregnant woman by court order, *Re F (in utero)*, 1988. The London Borough of Bromley claimed that the woman had a hippy lifestyle and suffered from mental health problems. It tried to make her foetus a ward of court. It sought a court order for her arrest, to force her into hospital for the remainder of her pregnancy. Bromley's goal was to take the baby into care when it was born. The court hearing was conducted in the woman's absence. The judge refused to intervene. Bromley appealed to the Court of Appeal, which also refused.

The three judges explained why English law should uphold a woman's autonomy. First, English case law did not recognize foetuses as separate legal entities until they were born. Therefore, foetuses could not be made wards of court. Second, the question whether pregnant women's civil liberties ought to be curtailed in this way was a matter for parliament and not for judges. Third, the judges thought that if foetuses could be made wards of court, this would create a most undesirable conflict. Ordinarily, in wardship cases, the welfare of the child is paramount. How could the welfare principle be reconciled with a pregnant woman's autonomy? *Re F (in utero)* has been followed in Canada. The Canadian Supreme Court rejected an attempt to take a pregnant glue-sniffer into protective custody for the sake of her foetus (*Winnipeg Child and Family Services* v G, 1997).

Despite this, court-ordered medical intervention against pregnant women enjoyed a temporary vogue in England in the 1990s. This was anomalous because, in English law, autonomy (the right to self-determination) is paramount. Every competent adult of sound mind is free to accept or to reject medical treatment, for reasons that are rational or irrational – or for no reason (*Sidaway*, 1985). To be competent means simply that a patient is capable of understanding the information which he or she is given, and of weighing it up to make a choice. If a patient is incapable of giving or withholding consent, the law requires doctors to act in the patient's best interests.

In 1993, the Court of Appeal upheld a court order by a judge authorizing treatment for an unconscious woman (*Re T*, 1993). T had an emergency Caesarean, following a car crash. While conscious, T had signed a form refusing blood. T was not a Jehovah's Witness. Complications arose and T became unconscious. Her family feared that T had been coerced by her mother, a staunch Jehovah's Witness, into signing the refusal form. A doctor initially told the judge, by telephone, that T was under the influence of pethidine and lacked capacity when she signed the form. The judge decided that T lacked capacity to refuse blood. Later, the doctor changed his evidence and said that T was capable of refusing after all, and the judge was forced to revise his ruling. He then concluded that T's refusal had not been a properly informed one in the circumstances. On appeal, Lord Donaldson stressed that, for an individual to defeat society's interest in saving life, he had to show that he exercised his choice to refuse treatment in clear terms. Lord Donaldson also commented that the only possible qualification to the principle of autonomy *might* be when a pregnant woman's choice might lead to the death of a viable foetus.

One practical lesson could have been learnt from T's case: the risk that, in hastily convened court hearings, judges might be misinformed about the facts. Unfortunately, this lesson was overlooked in a subsequent drift towards coerced obstetric intervention. Again, as in the US, once courts were eventually forced to consider the issues in detail, with full argument and evidence to hand, the women usually succeeded. However, it took time before women were allowed to argue their position fully. Initially, there was a rush to judgment.

A case heard in 1992 (*Re S*, 1993) was the first time that an English judge ordered a woman to have a Caesarean against her will. Mrs S was a Nigerian in labour in a London hospital. Her foetus was in a transverse lie and could not be born vaginally. Mrs S was capable of consenting, but opposed medical intervention. She wanted to let nature take its course. The hospital's lawyers applied to the President of the Family Division for a declaration authorizing non-consensual treatment. Mrs S had no chance to instruct lawyers or to be heard. The judge asked the Official Solicitor, a state official who usually appears for children in child welfare cases, or for unconscious patients, to appear as *amicus curiae* (friend of the court). The Official Solicitor instructed a QC. The hearing lasted about 20 minutes. The operation was said to be life-saving for both woman and foetus. The QC cited *Re AC*, 1990. He suggested that an American judge would order intervention. This was strange, because *Re AC*, 1990 upheld a pregnant woman's autonomy, even when the woman was near death.

In 1996, a number of cases received national attention. *Rochdale Health Care NHS Trust* v *Choudhury* (1996) concerned Mrs Choudhury, a Bangladeshi. She had had a previous bad experience of a consensual Caesarean section. When pregnant again in 1996, she was keen on a vaginal delivery. Late on a Friday afternoon, she was advised to have a Caesarean on the ground that her scar might rupture. She declined and signed a refusal form. This prompted a hasty application to the High Court in London. Mrs Choudhury was not represented. The hospital accepted that Mrs Choudhury was competent. The court was told that her uterus had already ruptured. Mr Justice Johnson authorized a non-consensual Caesarean. In fact, while the hearing was going on, Mrs Choudhury changed her mind and agreed to a Caesarean. The judge commented: 'So far as I know, no Judge has yet refused to make an order and has had to live with the subsequent news that a child has died that might have lived.' He then said: 'I am afraid the Judge has to do what some may call rough justice. I do not think there is a possibility of giving attention to the legal niceties' (Transcript 2, 4). In a written ruling produced later, the judge stated that Mrs Choudhury lacked capacity: she was unable to weigh up information to make a choice about anything, even of the most trivial kind, owing to the pain and stress of labour. In 1998, Mrs Choudhury had the order discharged and later settled an action for damages.

Mr Justice Johnston had been hearing another case, *Norfolk and Norwich Healthcare (NHS) Trust* v *W* (1997), when interrupted by the lawyer for Rochdale. The facts of this other case were that W had come into casualty and was found to be fully dilated, but in 'arrested labour'. W denied she was pregnant. A psychiatrist said that W was not suffering from a mental disorder and that she was capable of instructing a solicitor. However, W was not represented at court. The Official Solicitor again appeared as *amicus curiae*, using the same QC as in the case of Mrs S. He argued that, at common law, a judge could authorize the use of force on a patient who lacked the capacity to decide for herself whether to refuse treatment. Mr Justice Johnson ruled that W was unable to decide for herself, because she was unable to weigh up information to make a choice. He authorized the use of force to impose a forceps or Caesarean delivery.

Other reported cases in 1997 involved pregnant women who rejected Caesareans because of 'needle phobia', which the courts readily accepted as an incapacitating factor. One, *Re L* (1997), was heard in 22 minutes, in L's absence. Another case, *Re MB* (1997), was the first in which the woman was represented. A judge conducted the 'trial' by telephone late in the evening; it lasted barely half an hour. The judge declared that MB's needle phobia made her incapable of refusing anaesthesia. MB appealed. The Court of Appeal heard MB's appeal in the small hours. After midnight, it dismissed her appeal and ordered that force should be used to subdue her if necessary. Then, bizarrely, it directed the hospital to produce affidavit evidence and the lawyers to file written arguments. In its later written decision, the Court of Appeal stressed that, if MB were capable of deciding for herself, the court would have no jurisdiction to override her wishes.

St George's Healthcare NHS Trust v *S*, decided in May 1998, was the first successful challenge to a court-ordered Caesarean. The ruling convincingly affirms pregnant women's autonomy. In 1996, Ms S, a veterinary nurse, was eight months pregnant and suffering from pre-eclampsia. A local doctor advised her to go into hospital for bed-rest and to have her baby induced. S refused because she wanted a natural birth. She was then compulsorily detained under section 2 of the Mental Health Act 1983. This section authorizes compulsory detention where someone '*(a) ... is suffering from mental disorder of a nature or degree which warrants detention ... in a hospital for assessment (or for assessment followed by treatment) ... ; and (b) he ought to be so detained in the interests of his own safety or with a view to the protection of other persons'*. S was taken first to a mental hospital. Late at night she was transferred against her wishes to a maternity hospital, St George's. S explained her aversion to treatment clearly, both orally and in writing, and contacted solicitors the following day. S did not meet a consultant obstetrician until lunchtime. Their discussion focused on what drugs S might take to reduce her blood pressure.

At this time, and without her knowledge, St George's Hospital applied for a declaration from Mrs Justice Hogg that S should undergo non-consensual investigation, treatment and Caesarean surgery under 'agreed' anaesthetic. St George's accepted that S was capable of refusing treatment. The court was told, wrongly, that S had been in labour for 24 hours. The judge should have been told that S was not in labour, that she was only eight months pregnant and that she had instructed her own solicitors. When she finally saw the order, S was upset and queried it, in particular the reference to 'agreed' anaesthetic. She was sedated because she would not comply. Bizarrely, she was woken up some hours later and asked to consent to Caesarean surgery, which she again refused. Surgery was performed. When she came round the next morning, she rejected the baby and complained of assault. After S had recovered sufficiently from surgery, she was returned to the mental hospital, where she saw a consultant psychiatrist. He decided that she did not meet the criteria for detention under the Mental Health Act and she was discharged.

The Court of Appeal ruled that, although S was depressed, there was no basis for detaining her merely because she urgently needed treatment for pre-eclampsia, even though her opposition to treatment might appear unusual, or even bizarre (51). A lawful detention under the Mental Health Act has to be related or linked to mental disorder. It was flawed reasoning to assume that because S was non-compliant, she must have a mental disorder. But for her pre-eclampsia, the Court decided, 'there is nothing in the contemporaneous documents to suggest that an application for her detention would have been considered, let alone justified' (56). The Court noted that S was never offered any treatment for any mental disorder. It ruled that her detention was unlawful throughout. Even if she had been properly detained under the Mental Health Act, she could not have been compelled into medical procedures unconnected with her mental condition.

As for the court order, the Court of Appeal said, scathingly, 'The proceedings before Hogg J were so extraordinary and so unfortunate that we feel it appropriate to restate some fairly elementary points about declaratory relief' (58). It ruled that judges could not make declarations on an interim basis, but only after adequate investigation of the evidence put forward on either side. It pointed out that declarations, especially ones affecting personal autonomy, ought not to be made *ex parte* (that is, one side only appearing before the court). Apart from injustice and other more obvious objections, *ex parte* declarations could not protect medical and midwifery personnel from assault claims (62). The Court set aside Mrs Justice Hogg's order, enabling S to recover substantial damages. Its decision meant that all court orders made previously, in cases where women were unrepresented, had no legal effect.

St George's argued that the principle of the sanctity of life could be used to override S's autonomy. The Court of Appeal responded that 'a forced invasion of a competent adult's body against her will even for the most laudable of motives (the preservation of life)' could not be ordered, without irremediably damaging the principle of self-determination. It stressed the importance of protecting individual autonomy, particularly when the motive for interfering with it might seem commendable. As for the foetus, the Court of Appeal said that it was human, but not a separate person from its mother. Even though pregnancy increased a pregnant woman's personal responsibilities, 'it does not diminish her entitlement to decide whether or not to undergo medical treatment' (50). The Court reasoned that if a foetus could be benefited by way of court-ordered treatment, against a pregnant woman's wishes, then the principle of autonomy would be annihilated. Its approach was gender-neutral, and a resounding affirmation of liberal individualism:

medical science will no doubt advance to the stage when a very minor procedure undergone by an adult would save the life of his or her child, or perhaps the child of a complete stranger ... If, however, the adult were compelled to agree, or rendered helpless to desist, the principle of autonomy would be extinguished. (47)

Arguments in favour of foetal rights continue. In a talk to the Medico-Legal Society in London, the lawyer who represented the hospitals in the cases of W and MB, mentioned above, presented a talk entitled 'Should the Foetus have Rights in Law?' (Grace, 1999). The talk concentrated on forced Caesareans. He began by posing the question: 'In the medico-legal context, to what extent can or should the fetus, the unborn child (let's call it what it is), be protected against an irresponsible mother who doesn't have her child's best interests at heart?' He summarized three possible justifications for limiting pregnant women's rights to self-determination, at least in the case of a term foetus. One is that a woman who has chosen not to abort owes a duty to 'the human being that she has chosen to bear'. The second is that the public interest requires the birth of children free from avoidable harm, on grounds of both morality and the high cost of disability to society. The third is the public interest in the integrity of the medical profession, since many obstetricians believe that the pregnant woman is two patients.

These arguments echo those used by foetal rights proponents in the US. But it is hard to see how a woman's decision not to have an abortion means that she forfeits her right to bodily integrity. It does, however, suggest that pregnant women are expected to be self-sacrificing. I suspect that this argument really operates at the level of emotion, rather than logic. As the Court of Appeal pointed out in the case of S, if an adult can be compelled to forfeit her autonomy for the sake of a foetus, then logically adults could be forcibly operated on to save the child of a complete stranger. If only pregnant woman were forced to give up their autonomy, it would mean that pregnant women are less equal than, and foetuses are superior to, everybody else!

It is also hard to see how moral or economic imperatives could justify the forcible treatment of pregnant women, but not of other groups in society. Foetuses, unlike children, are located inside women's bodies, and avoiding harm to a foetus may involve physical harm to the woman. Ordinarily, our society does not require that people be forcibly harmed in order to benefit others. If a person agrees voluntarily to undergo harm for another's sake, this is regarded as praiseworthy, even heroic. Whilst women usually go to considerable lengths to ensure that they produce healthy babies, they are not penalized for giving birth to dead or disabled ones. Nor are women required to abort disabled foetuses. If society considered that disabled people represented an unacceptable burden, it could require that all disabled foetuses be aborted.

Will the Human Rights Act 1998 change anything? The Act gives effect to certain fundamental rights laid down in the European Convention for the Protection of Human Rights (1950). Article 8 guarantees the right to respect for private life. This Article includes the right to physical and moral integrity. At the time of writing, the courts are adopting a cautious approach to the new Act. It seems unlikely that it could be used to take away pregnant women's civil liberties. The Act is not intended to take away pre-existing freedoms. Therefore, if a challenge to pregnant women's autonomy is made under the new Act, it is probable that English courts will uphold the status quo. The main lesson to be learnt from the English experience, to date, is that legal processes can be used successfully in counteracting threats to women's autonomy in reproductive decision-making.

List of cases

US cases

Roe v *Wade* 410 US 113 (1973).
Thornburgh v *American College of Gynecologists* 476 US 747 (1986).
Re AC 533 A.2d 611 (1987); 573 A 2d 1235 (1990).
Planned Parenthood v *Casey* 505 US 833 (1992).
Re Doe 632 NE 2d 326 (1994).
Whitner v *State* 492 SE 2d 777 (1997).
State of Wisconsin ex rel. Angela MW v *Kruzicki* 561 NW 2d 729 (1997).
Fetus Brown 689 NE 2d 397 (1997).
Ferguson v *City of Charleston*, Supreme Court of the United States, 21 March 2001.

Canadian cases

Winnipeg Child and Family Services v *G* (1997) 3 BHRC 611.

UK cases

Sidaway v *Bethlem Royal Hospital* [1985] AC 871.
F (in utero) [1988] Fam 122.
Re F [1990] 2 AC 1.
Burton v *Islington Health Authority* [1993] QB 204.
Re S [1993] Fam 123.
Re T [1993] Fam 95.
Rochdale Healthcare NHS Trust v *Choudhury* [1997] 1 FCR 274. Transcript of official court tape recording by Barnett, Lenton & Co. (1997).
Norwich and Norfolk Healthcare NHS Trust v *W* [1997] 1 FCR 269.
Re L [1997] 2 FLR 837.
Re MB [1997] 2 FCR 541.
AG's Reference (No. 3 of 1994) [1998] AC 245.
St George's Healthcare NHS Trust v *S* [1999] Fam 26.

Further reading

Harris, J., *The Value of Life: An Introduction to Medical Ethics* (London: Routledge, 1985).

Lublin, N., *Pandora's Box: Feminism Confronts Reproductive Technology* (New York: Rowman and Littlefield, 1998).

Richards, J.R., *The Sceptical Feminist: A Philosophical Enquiry* (Harmondsworth: Penguin, 1994).

Rowland, R., *Living Laboratories: Women and Reproductive Technology* (London: Lime Tree, 1993).

9
Long-term Psychological Effects of Child Sexual Abuse

Gillian Oaker

Introduction

One outcome of the consciousness-raising groups within the women's movement in the 1960s and 1970s was the recognition that many women had experienced childhood sexual abuse. Increased awareness and dialogue began to change the *Zeitgeist*, so that mental health services in particular were forced to acknowledge that this experience was not fantasy, but a cruel reality for many adult women (Rosenfeld et al., 1979; Surrey et al., 1990), more recently enabling men with similar experiences to speak about them.

The past decade has produced a plethora of literature, media coverage and psychological research into the effects of such sexual abuse. A substantial body of knowledge now demonstrates that a history of childhood sexual abuse can have long-term psychological effects for some, but not all, adult women with these experiences (Beitchman et al., 1992; Cahill et al., 1991; Finkelhor, 1984; Gold et al., 1996; Gregory-Bills and Rhodeback, 1995; Ross-Gower et al., 1998; Ussher and Dewberry, 1995). Commonly reported effects include depression, anxiety, fear of men, substance abuse, low self-esteem and sexual difficulties (Cahill et al., 1991). However, the research literature is not consistent on what leads to such difficulties. Some authors suggest that repeated and prolonged abuse leads to poorer mental health (Bagley and Ramsey, 1986; Russell, 1986; Ussher and Dewberry, 1995) while others contradict this assertion (Courtois, 1979; Finkelhor, 1979). The literature review by Faust et al. (1995), suggests that stepfathers are more likely than other family members to commit incest and that more clinical psychopathology and adjustment problems arise for those abused by a family member. Others argue that a broader view of the context and nature of the abuse is more fruitful than a narrow focus on one relationship, in explaining why only some people experience long term difficulties (Ussher and Dewberry, 1995).

Cognitive therapy and childhood sexual abuse

The literature progresses from describing the behavioural components of the abuse (Bagley and Ramsey, 1986) to the family and developmental context (Alexander, 1992; Cole and Putman, 1992) to the meaning, or cognitive appraisal an individual attaches to such an experience (Mullen et al., 1996; Ussher and Dewberry, 1995). In particular, the coercive statements the abuser makes to the child seem to have an impact on the development of the child's belief system (Ussher and Dewberry, 1995). This view complements the use of cognitive therapy (Briere, 1992; Jehu, 1988) to address the effects of such abuse. Cognitive therapy emphasizes identifying, examining and evaluating thoughts and beliefs about self and the world – often called 'core beliefs' or 'schemas' (Beck, 1967) – and how they influence mood and behaviour (Beck, 1976; 1991; 1995). An integral element here is the collaborative nature of the therapeutic relationship, where the therapist and the patient work together to understand the development and impact of a particular belief system. This helps equalize the power relationship between clinician and patient and increases empowerment, mutual respect and self-knowledge.

Childhood sexual abuse can have far-reaching effects on a woman's beliefs about herself as a person, the world, people in general and, consequently, her different roles in life. The use of the 'core beliefs' model, the collaborative approach and the concept that the statements made by the abuser may be influential suggests that cognitive therapy could be a useful treatment.

The cognitive therapy approach to treatment is well documented for a variety of disorders including depression, panic disorder, obsessional compulsive disorder and post-traumatic stress disorder (Clark and Fairburn, 1997). As with any psychotherapeutic intervention, developing a formulation is a key aspect of the intervention. A formulation is the term used to describe a general model, or framework, which helps patient and therapist understand why and how certain difficulties have arisen (Freeman, 1992; Persons, 1989). For some adults who have experienced childhood sexual abuse, there can be complex presenting problems and the formulation acts not only as a guide to the treatment process, but also allows the containment and understanding of seemingly overwhelming emotional states. A fundamental aspect of my practice as a clinical psychologist is to help the person understand that many of their responses are, in fact, normal responses to an abnormal situation.

While identifying a history of sexual abuse is not a diagnosis, unlike a formal mental 'illness', none the less such a history can lead to long-term difficulties. By incorporating the theoretical notions of cognitive therapy, schema development (Young, 1990) and schema change (Padesky, 1994) in the evolution of a belief system, the therapist and the woman can jointly figure out what led to her difficulties and develop strategies to help reduce their negative impact.

The following case is one example from my clinical practice of how cognitive therapy is used to address long-term difficulties which may be experienced by women following childhood sexual abuse.

The following details are published with the person's permission, with significant details omitted and amended to maintain her anonymity and privacy.

Case description: Mary

Mary, a 34-year-old woman, was referred for treatment by her family doctor when she disclosed that a male relative sexually abused her as a child.

Mary was married with three children. She visited the doctor's surgery up to five times a week with her asthmatic youngest child. Mary had been treated with anti-depressant medication on six separate occasions with minimal effect. Mary was a quiet, apologetic and extremely self-deprecating woman, who could not easily articulate her difficulties.

Assessment

Each weekly therapy session lasted an hour. The first three sessions were spent collecting a detailed description of the affective, behavioural and cognitive aspects of her difficulties, as well as a full family, social and medical history. The issue of confidentiality and therapeutic boundaries were explicitly discussed, only to be breached if she informed the therapist of harm to a child or herself. The boundaries of the therapeutic relationship were clearly outlined, as all people who have been sexually abused have experienced a direct violation of relationship boundaries.

Family background

Mary, the eldest of five children, described her upbringing as emotionally and economically deprived. She remembered her father as moody and her mother as emotionally distant. Both parents worked in low-paid, labour-intensive, rural occupations. She recalled that the family was often ostracized and marginalized by the local community, this being exacerbated by resentment at the children's receiving free school meals.

Between the age of five and eleven, an adult male relative had sexually abused Mary. When she told her parents, their response was to say she should avoid contact with him – impossible when he was a frequent visitor to the family home.

Two significant events led Mary to seek help. First, attending a family event when she saw that relative and heard him use a particular phrase she associated with the abuse. Second, in the same week, one of her children brought home a science project which reminded her how the offender would seek her out on her return from school and inquire about her schoolwork. Her child's science project was the same as one she herself had completed at that age and which she associated with the first episode of sexual abuse.

Presenting problems

Mary's main presenting problems were panic disorder, obsessional compulsive disorder, depression, social phobia and episodes of flashbacks and nightmares.

1. *Panic disorder.* Mary had a moderate level of anxiety with a Beck Anxiety Inventory (BAI) score of 27 (Beck et al., 1988) and she experienced up to ten panic attacks a week. She interpreted any physical symptom, such as headaches, sweating, dizziness, breathing difficulty and shaking, as clear evidence of a catastrophic illness. These thoughts often arose in response to concerns about her youngest child's health or social events. The panic attacks often resulted in seeking reassurance from her doctor, then feeling angry with herself, guilt and using cleaning rituals to reduce the overwhelming emotions.
2. *Obsessional compulsive disorder.* Mary described a range of obsessional compulsive behaviours. Whenever she experienced strong emotions she would use cleaning rituals to calm herself. She believed that if she, and the house, were completely clean, then all her problems would be solved. The beliefs associated with this behaviour included 'If I'm not clean then I am bad', 'I am dirty' and

'If everything is clean, no harm will come to me or my children'. The relief was only short-lived and had become increasingly complex and labour intensive.

3. *Depression.* Mary was asked to complete the Beck Depression Inventory (Beck et al., 1961). The score was 44, indicating a clinically significant level of severe depression. She believed that she was a useless mother and wife. When experiencing a low mood, she interpreted this as evidence of her stupidity and lack of self-control. Underpinning her negative thoughts about herself was a strongly held assumption that 'If I show my feelings then I'll lose complete control and lose everything'. Two aspects of her history had encouraged this belief. First, her parents rarely responded to emotional distress; and any response was often punitive, telling her not to be so stupid. Second, the abuser said that if she told, everyone would think she was mad.

4. *Social phobia.* At the time Mary sought treatment, she was avoiding most social situations, including collecting the children from school, shopping and family gatherings. She believed that she could not trust people and that if she felt strong emotions she would lose control.

5. *Flashbacks and nightmares.* Mary was experiencing flashbacks on a daily basis. This is often described as feeling oneself as being back in time, re-experiencing the same sensations, emotions and images. These were often triggered by particular smells, especially male sweat. She described nightmares of 'being trapped' and she often awoke, sweating, with palpitations and chest pains.

The initial focus of a cognitive therapy assessment is to gather information on the automatic thoughts and behaviours associated with difficulties happening in the person's everyday life. A 'map' or formulation can then be developed to link the background history and the belief system and indicate treatment options, clarifying 'How did I get here and how do I get out of here?' In this case, a diagrammatic formulation was developed from the assessment material (see Figure 9.1) and amended as therapy progressed and additional information was discovered.

Intervention and treatment

As Mary was experiencing several difficulties, we decided to prioritize the problem list. As the panic disorder had the greatest impact on her day-to-day life, we decided this would be our initial focus. The panic

Figure 9.1   Cognitive Therapy Formulation for Mary

Early Experience ↓	Father, moody and distant. Mother emotionally distant. Economic deprivation, social isolation. Family rule: 'Don't speak about how you feel'. Sexual abuse 5–11 years, told by offender 'No one will believe you if you tell'.
Core beliefs (schemas) ↓	'I am dirty and bad. I am powerless. I am stupid. People are dangerous, you can't trust them. The world is unsafe.'
Assumptions (rules for living) ↓	'If I show my feelings then I'll lose control and lose everything. If I tell people what happened, they won't believe me. If I'm not clean, I am bad. I must be on my guard all the time.'
Critical Incident(s) ↓	Family event, meeting offender, use of specific phrase. Child returning home with science project.
Negative Automatic Thoughts	'I don't deserve help. I shouldn't be feeling like this. I must be clean. I've got cancer. I'm demented. Everyone thinks I'm mad, they don't believe me.'
Affect	Panic, depression, guilt, anger.
Cognitive	Catastrophization, overgeneralization, selective abstraction.
Behavioural	Avoidance, withdrawal, cleaning.
Somatic	Chest pains, dizziness, palpitations, breathlessness, sweating, headaches, insomnia and nausea.

model (Clark, 1986; 1988), which demonstrates how individuals can interpret bodily sensations catastrophically, is easily understood by patients, serving as a straightforward introduction to the basic tenets of the cognitive approach. Using this was the primary focus of the first six sessions.

Initially, Mary was asked to keep a diary of when the panic attacks occurred, noting down the situation, bodily reactions and cognitions, or thoughts, and behaviours at the time. This excerpt from session 4 demonstrates how such cognitive distortions are addressed.

Therapist: Can you give me an example of a recent situation that was associated with a panic attack?

Mary: Well, I was cleaning the kitchen and it wasn't helping.

T: When you say it wasn't helping, what do you mean?

M: I had a headache and it wasn't going away.

T: So, what's so bad about having a headache?

M: I don't know.

T: Let's write this down. You are cleaning the kitchen and the first thought you have is 'This isn't helping the headache to go away'. Was anything else going through your mind?

M: Well ... there must be something serious, for it to be so bad.

T: Good, so another thought was 'It must be something serious'. What would be serious?

M: Umm ... it might be a brain tumour or something. I know I'm pathetic, it's stupid.

T: OK, so another thought is that it might mean you had a brain tumour. Say that was true, what would be so bad about that?

M: I would die and leave my children. (*starts crying*)

T: That's a very painful thought. What would it mean to you if you should die and leave your children?

M: They would be all alone and in danger. No one to look after them and protect them.

These are examples of activating core beliefs that 'the world is unsafe', 'other people are dangerous' and 'I am powerless and stupid'. It is also apparent that Mary's own experience of abandonment in childhood strongly influences her beliefs about her role as a mother. These are also linked to Mary's fears for her own health.

T: That thought has triggered off a lot of strong feelings. Am I right?

M: Yes. (*a look of relief on her face*)

T: Let's try to look at the evidence and see whether the thought is completely true. What do we have, to say that you do have a brain tumour?

M: I've got a headache.

T: Yes, any other evidence?

M: I feel dizzy sometimes.

T:	Does that always correspond with a headache?
M:	No ... not always. Sometimes I feel dizzy when I'm waiting for the kids after school.
T:	Umm, that's interesting. So, the evidence we have so far for a brain tumour is having a headache and feeling dizzy – anything else?
M:	No, I can't think of anything.
T:	OK, what evidence do we have that it might *not* be a brain tumour?
M:	I don't know.
T:	How might we try to figure this out?
M:	Well. I suppose Dr. X [family doctor] would know.
T:	Yes, we could ask Dr. X ...

At this point I am mindful of trying to help Mary to reduce her contact with her family doctor (GP) without contradicting her, which would make her think she was stupid.

T:	Is there anywhere else we could get this information from? Have you ever known anyone with a brain tumour?
M:	No, not really, but there was someone on 'Casualty' [popular television medical drama] last week.
T:	Tell me about that.
M:	Well this woman had a brain tumour and she had a headache and was dizzy.
T:	Anything else?
M:	(*smiles*) Oh, I see what you're getting at. Yes, she had lost her sight and had had a fit and couldn't speak properly.
T:	So what do you think we're getting at?
M:	That if I had a brain tumour I would have other symptoms.
T:	Why don't we try the same approach with the thought about the children being all alone?

By gently and carefully beginning to practise cognitive restructuring, by looking at a thought and seeking evidence for and against it, we can focus on a slightly less emotive belief before moving on to more emotionally-laden beliefs. Consequently, Mary starts to gain a sense of competence and to experience and articulate her emotions. She would have found starting with the most emotionally-laden belief very difficult, as her coping strategy is to avoid strong emotions, following the family rule. If she had avoided this exercise it would have further confirmed to her that she was stupid.

Mary was encouraged by this approach. Between sessions she began to record similar situations and challenges to the catastrophic thoughts by looking at the evidence for and against. By the end of session 6, the frequency of the panic attacks had reduced to two a week and the BAI score had dropped to 15. Her contact with the GP had been reduced to once a fortnight. This work carried on in parallel with the next phase, sessions 7 to 15, which addressed the obsessional compulsive behaviour.

This behaviour arose from two strongly held beliefs, 'If I don't clean, then something awful will happen' and 'If I'm dirty, then I'm bad'. The cleaning behaviour helped her, in the short term, to feel less anxious, angry and depressed. But, soon after, she would experience these feelings again, which led to an increase in the behaviour until, ultimately, she became increasingly depressed.

The first stage of the intervention was for Mary to note down the situations that preceded the cleaning behaviour, and associated thoughts. This record showed that she was spending up to six hours a day cleaning the kitchen and bathroom. It is worth noting that the sexual abuse occurred in these rooms in the parental home, hence their particular significance. An experiment was agreed that Mary would try to reduce the cleaning behaviour by five minutes and see what thoughts and feelings arose.

An excerpt from session 9 describes some of the challenges to her thinking.

T:	I see from your diary that you have tried to reduce your cleaning.
M:	Yes.
T:	How have you found this?
M:	Hard.
T:	Shall we go through one of the situations?
M:	If you want.

Mary's short, curt answers clearly indicate a reluctance and irritation with this approach. This is a good indication that she is beginning to feel safe enough in the sessions to express other emotions apart from passivity and I am hoping that she will be able to say this directly to me.

T:	So, you decided to reduce the time cleaning the kitchen by ten minutes on Monday. When you thought about doing this, what went through your mind?
M:	I can't do it.
T:	How did that make you feel?
M:	There's no point carrying on with it.
T:	Hmm, so another thought. And what was the emotion attached to these thoughts?
M:	Pissed off.
T:	That's interesting. Can you tell me a bit more? What was making you pissed off?
M:	I thought I can't do this. (*looks away*) Gill's making me do this, she'll be angry with me if I don't do it.
T:	Mm … Some powerful thoughts. 'I can't do this' and then that Gill was making you do this and that Gill would be angry. Can you remember the first time *ever* you had these thoughts?
M:	(*long pause and quiet voice*) If I didn't do what Z [male relative] said, he would get angry. (*resumes eye contact*)
T:	So we can begin to see how these beliefs might have developed. But say I was angry with you, what would be so bad about that?
M:	I couldn't cope and you'd stop seeing me.
T:	That's interesting. Where does that belief come from, that if you show what you feel you will be left?
M:	Well, Mum and Dad, I suppose.
T:	Can you give me an example?
M:	If any of us were hurt they would ignore us. Like my brother fell off this wall and it was obvious something was wrong because he cried, but Mum just told him not to be such a cry-baby and it wasn't until he went to school that the teacher told Mum to take him to the doctor and his arm was broken.
T:	So we have another example of the family rule. If you show feelings you will be ignored. Have you cried here?
M:	Yes.
T:	And what happened?
M:	We talked it through and you listened.
T:	So what does that tell you?
M:	You don't ignore me.

This example demonstrates how certain beliefs and rules have developed and the beginning of challenging those beliefs within the session. Mary is starting to learn that not all people ignore the feelings of others and, following on, that there may be alternative ways to deal with her emotions, as shown below:

T:	Yes. Let's look at the other emotion you mentioned: anger. What would be so bad if you were angry with me?
M:	I couldn't.
T:	What do you think would happen if you were angry?
M:	I'd completely lose it.
T:	How?
M:	I'd go mad and I'd end up in A [psychiatric hospital].
T:	What else might happen, bearing in mind what we've done when you cried?
M:	We might talk about it (*looking wary*)
T:	Yes we could do that, shall we give it a go?
M:	OK.

This dialogue also highlights how to differentiate between feeling anger and a justifiable irritation in being told what to do. Anger is a healthy emotion in response to her experience, and the aim is to help express this in a manner safe for her. By practising assertive strategies within and between sessions, Mary began to learn that her worst fears were not realized and she could reduce her need to clean. Not all the responses were positive, as her husband, in particular, found the more assertive Mary confusing. At one point he said she should see a psychiatrist as she was obviously mad. Prior to therapy, Mary would have wholeheartedly accepted this view, but in utilizing the cognitive therapy approach she was able to explore the evidence for and against this idea and explain to her husband her reasons for saying no on some occasions.

The predominant theme of the cleaning behaviour was to prevent the experience and expression of strong emotions. By reducing the time spent cleaning, easier access to these thoughts and feelings was possible. The use of cognitive strategies, assertive techniques and talking with female friends about how they dealt with strong emotions helped to increase her repertoire of coping strategies, such as using her diary to write down how she was feeling, and checking out whether her beliefs always came true.

The second belief, 'I am dirty, therefore I am bad', was strongly linked with her depressed mood and an extensive bathing ritual. This became the primary focus of the next few sessions. The core belief, or schema, 'I am bad' is a commonly held belief amongst many of the adults I see, who have been sexually abused in childhood. The offender had told Mary that the abuse was her fault, with such phrases as 'You're making me do this' and that, if she told, no one would believe her and anyway they would think she was mad. Part of this came true as her parents did not act on her disclosure of the abuse; furthermore, being referred to see a clinical psychologist initially served to confirm, that she must be mad. She grew up believing all of the statements made by the offender (see Ussher and Dewberry, 1995) and interpreted many of her actions, thoughts and feelings using this template.

The use of the formulation enabled Mary to understand how she had developed these beliefs, and the intervention thus far showed that they might not be entirely true. Until this point, the focus had been on the here and now, the panic attacks, the cleaning rituals as responses to her beliefs and the associated emotions; attention was now paid to schemas or core beliefs.

Mary was able to describe in more detail how the belief 'I am dirty, therefore I am bad' arose from particular sexual behaviours performed by the offender. During these episodes she felt bad and, therefore, in her child's mind she thought 'If I feel bad, it must mean I am bad'. Children inevitably label emotions simplistically and the term 'bad' can encompass a range of different emotions. She knew objectively she was not dirty, but would often say 'But I still feel bad'. This exemplifies the dilemma that can arise in cognitive therapy when the patient will say 'I know it up here', pointing to their head, 'but I don't feel it here' pointing to their heart.

Mary developed confidence in the standard methods of diary-keeping, logical analysis and searching for alternative interpretations using Socratic questioning – using a series of questions and discussions to help examine alternative views. A further skill was added to her repertoire, that of how to modify core beliefs or schemas using a continuum method (Padesky, 1994; Padesky and Greenberger, 1995). This is a diagrammatic representation of extreme beliefs demonstrated in the next section.

T: How would you like to be, if you weren't bad?
M: Just OK.
T: Can you tell me the characteristics of a 'bad' person?

M: Well, they'd be cruel, uncaring, violent.
T: So do you use these words to judge yourself?
M: Yes. Well, sometimes.
T: Let's make a scale of these points. (Drawing three lines
        and labelling one end 0 per cent and the other 100 per
        cent). So we have three characteristics of a bad person. At
        one end we have always cruel to everyone and at the
        other we have never cruel to anyone and similarly for the
        other two. Can you put a cross on the each line using this
        measurement to show where you would put yourself?
T: What do you notice about these crosses?
M: I seem to use the caring one more to judge myself.

Figure 9.2   Diagrammatic representation of Mary's core beliefs about herself

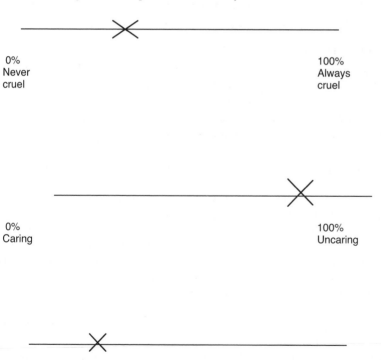

0%   100%
Never   Always
cruel   cruel

0%   100%
Caring   Uncaring

0%   100%
Never violent   Always violent

T:	Yes, that's interesting isn't it? It fits with many of the judgements you have made about yourself as a mother. So what do you make of the others?
M:	(*pause*) Maybe I'm not all bad.
T:	Maybe not. Another way we can look at this is to keep what's called a positive data log. Sometimes when we have very strong beliefs it's like having very strong views or prejudices about other people, the world or ourselves. So, what I suggest is you begin to look for evidence over the next few weeks to see if you're an OK person, no matter how small.

This intervention helped Mary to see that her belief about herself may not be 100 per cent true and there might be an alternative way for her to view herself. This part of therapy can last for several weeks, as more evidence is gathered to challenge the belief, and for the client to rate how much they believe each new and old schema.

End of therapy

Mary and I met for a total of 28 sessions. At the final follow-up session, Mary was no longer depressed or clinically anxious, the Beck Depression Inventory score was 5 and the Beck Anxiety Inventory score was 8. Her cleaning rituals had reduced to a manageable level and she was actively involved in many social activities.

Conclusion

This case study has demonstrated that the long-term impact of child sexual abuse can be understood and treated using a well-recognized and validated form of psychotherapy. By actively working together in partnership, Mary and I were able to develop a clear map and explore a range of different routes to help her to find a way out of her maze. This approach enabled a woman, within the safety of the therapy, to become stronger and more confident and for mutual respect to develop.

For generations, women have been seen as 'hysterical', 'manipulative' and 'histrionic' by a Western, male-dominated psychiatry, when they simply wanted to tell their story and to be understood. To do this and to find ways of dealing with extremely strong emotions, they have sometimes had to go to extreme and risky lengths, such as self-injury and self-harm using drugs, alcohol and overdoses. Now the *Zeitgeist* is changing as more women are working in health and social care agencies, more children are being protected and more adults are enabled to rebuild their lives as their stories are listened to. More creative and innovative models of treatment can only be developed if we listen to each other and continue the sharing of knowledge. Some of the rigid professional barriers are already dissolving within interdisciplinary clinical practice. As such power structures crumble, some practitioners are learning that sharing knowledge and experience leads to a greater diversity and richness of therapeutic practice. This can only be of benefit to women service users.

Further reading

Ainscough, C. and Toon, K., *Breaking Free* (London: Sheldon Press, 2000).

Butler, G., *Manage Your Mind* (Oxford: Oxford University Press, 1995).

Gold, S.N., Hughes, D.M. and Swingle, J.M., 'Characteristics of Childhood Sexual Abuse among Female Survivors in Therapy', *Child Abuse and Neglect* 20 (1996) 323–35.

Greenberger, D. and Padesky, C., *Mind over Mood. Change How You Feel by Changing How You Think* (New York: Guilford Press, 1996).

10
Maternal Depression and the Needs of the Child

Anne Greig And Dawn Gregory

Introduction

Depression is a highly prevalent condition which ranges from mild, temporary mood distress to severe, persistent symptoms which impair normal functioning. In its worst form it kills. It has been reported as occurring twice as frequently in women as in men, and more in women with babies and young children (American Psychiatric Association, 1987).

The association between maternal depression and adverse outcomes in children has been widely researched and usefully reviewed by Downey and Coyne (1990). However, much remains unexplored about the nature of maternal depression and about the long-term consequences for the child. A depressed woman with a baby or young child may have been depressed for many years, or for a shorter period during her pregnancy, or for physiological, social or psychological reasons since giving birth. A child may exhibit disturbed or anxious behaviour or other forms of 'abnormal' physical or emotional development for a variety of reasons of which maternal depression is likely to be one (for example, Campbell, Cohn and Meyers, 1995; Hammen, 1999). These manifestations may be temporary and non-harmful in the long term, or they may constitute the roots of problems which, if untreated, persist into adolescence and adulthood. A recent study, looking at child outcomes at five years old, suggests that high levels of severity and chronicity of maternal depression were significant in relation to behaviour problems and low vocabulary scores (Brennan et al., 2000). However, little is known about developmental effects beyond this age.

Furthermore, the training, policy and practice guidelines which form the framework for care professional interaction with a depressed mother and disturbed child tend to be responsive only to one or other of these individuals. This results in a piecemeal and often professionally isolated approach, rather than working with their joint needs and with the problem as a whole, during the critical early stages of their developing relationship. However, it is not simple to provide health and social care services which are appropriate and effective in this multi-client context, across the wide-ranging spectra of both maternal depression and infant behaviour disturbance and within a constrained professional framework.

This chapter reviews theory and research surrounding the nature and causes of maternal depression, its effects on mother and child and on their relationship with the outside world. It goes on to report a research study exploring the views and experiences of involved health and social care professionals and identifying some obstacles inhibiting access to appropriate resources and services (Gregory, 1997). It concludes by making recommendations for a more integrated form of planning and service provision.

Theoretical perspectives on maternal depression

As the introduction suggests, depression is a wide-ranging condition which cannot be viewed as a homogeneous phenomenon. Broadly speaking, it may be viewed as either primarily biological or primarily psychological. Clearly the values and health beliefs of professionals working in this field will be crucial in determining the type of help or treatment that is provided. Thus it is important to consider the relevance of related theories of depression to their potential application by practitioners.

Biological theories of depression include those relating to genetic transmission and to physiological disturbance. Research findings from family, twin and adoption studies indicate that genetic factors contribute to affective disorders including depression, but the mode of transmission for such a heterogeneous condition has not, so far, been possible to identify (McGuffin and Sargeant, 1991). Physiological disturbance focuses on the body's neurochemical, endocrine and limbic systems which support its controlling and communicating functions. If any of these systems begins to fluctuate or malfunction, affective disorders such as depression may result. As with the genetic or 'heredity' argument, origins and connections have been difficult to isolate, leading to the conclusion that depression is too complex a phenomenon for it to be satisfactorily explained by any one single biological factor (Baldessarini, 1985; Schwartz and Schwartz, 1993).

Thus, while physiological factors affecting hormonal activity during adolescence, pregnancy, childbirth, menstruation and the menopause are frequently cited, it is rarely possible to attribute any of these as a sole cause of maternal depression. In particular, studies of postpartum or postnatal depression have been inconclusive, supporting the view that the explanation for higher rates of depression in women is likely to be located in the interplay between genetic transmission, female endocrine physiology and psychosocial factors (Weissman and Klerman, 1985).

Longstanding psychological theories of relevance to maternal depression include: Freud's view of it as hostility turned inwards (Freud, 1917); behaviourists' views of it as learned behaviour (for example, Skinner, 1953) and socio-cultural conditioning (Seligman, 1974); and Beck's notions of cognitive distortion and dysfunctional information processing (Beck, 1976; 1991). Beck identifies three interactive faulty cognitive schemata that characterize depression: a negative view of the self, of the current situation and of the future.

Sociological theories which may impact on individual women's psychological perceptions include: labelling theory, which constructs women as subject to more social sanctions, more prone to be labelled as mentally ill and, thereby liable to social control interventions (Sheppard, 1991); and feminism, which locates maternal depression within the stress and isolation experienced by mothers due to low structural and cultural status and support (Evans, 1995).

Brown and Harris (1978) studied the major life-events and difficulties that characterize the lives of depressed and well women. They identified several risk factors which make depression more likely: having three or more young children; lack of an intimate and confiding partner; lack of paid employment outside the home; and loss of the mother before the age of eleven. Most single mothers tend to experience more than one of these depressogenic conditions (Brockington and Kumar, 1982). These findings emphasize the complexity which surrounds the origins of maternal depression.

The foregoing theoretical and research perspectives on the causes of maternal depression and associated potentials for diagnosis and treatment are thus neither exhaustive nor mutually exclusive. They inform a range of approaches when undertaking clinical, social and psychosocial assessments of family circumstances where maternal depression is a feature. A comprehensive understanding of these perspectives, and how they may interact, increases the potential for developing a more holistic approach to supporting depressed mothers and their children. First, however, it is necessary to explore further the impact of depression not only upon mothers, but also upon their children.

The effect of maternal depression upon mother and child in the early years

The experience of depression can be conveyed in the often metaphorical expressions mothers use to describe their feelings and perceptions. In research on depressed mothers and their relationships with their pre-school children, the restrictions of motherhood have been described thus:

> It's like living in a glass jar and I just can't get out.

> I ... search ... searching for the light at the end of this long, dark tunnel.

> I dance in the kitchen, you know, I lock her [the child] out, turn up the music as loud as I can and I dance, dance or scream.
>> (Previously unpublished quotes from ongoing research;
>> see Greig and Howe, 2001)

Depressed mothers exhibit symptoms which can impair cognitive, emotional, behavioural and physical functioning (World Health Organization, 1992). Their thinking is characterized by low self-esteem, negative self-perception and low confidence in parenting ability. Other problems with thinking include poor memory, concentration and marked negativity of thought in general.

The child of a mother affected in this way may not receive the consistent, alert attention and positive involvement which children draw upon naturally for reassurance and guidance. Flat emotional expression, sadness, irritability and hostility may form the core emotional experience of the depressed mother and her child so that the full range of healthy emotional experience is not encountered. The child may not, therefore, receive the kind of reciprocal, positive, playful interaction, which serves so well to modulate emotional arousal or experience a positive resolution of anxiety through parental attunement. This is a particular risk with severe post-natal depression (Cox, Puckering et al., 1987; Murray and Trevarthen, 1991; Murray, 1992). During the first five years, the child has to accomplish many developmental tasks for effective cognitive, emotional and social functioning. Socially, the child needs to achieve attachment to the mother and independence, good relationships with peers and siblings, and the ability to play socially and collaboratively with others. Cognitively, the child needs to develop communicative competence, imaginative play and an understanding of the thoughts, intentions and feelings of self and others. Emotionally, the child needs to achieve regulation of arousal and appropriate expression of emotional states and prosocial behaviour. In the early years, the attainment of these developmental tasks is mediated by psychological processes and mechanisms which, in this period of rapid formation, are vulnerable to interpersonal influences.

Impaired bonding processes and mechanisms can disrupt the child's ability to form a secure attachment pattern. An insecure attachment can lead to the development of an insecure internal working model and, in turn, to low expectations of themselves and others (Bowlby, 1991). Positive attachment requires sensitive attunement by the mother to the infant and is achieved through a cycle of arousal and relaxation and positive, reciprocal interaction between the mother and the infant. These processes form the crucial foundation of early mother–infant communication and are vital for establishing bonds, routines, scaffolding of experience and the regulation of emotion (Murray and Trevarthen, 1991).

The socio-cognitive world of the young child is compromised when the mother is depressed. The child is heavily dependent on her for interpreting emotional experiences and intellectual events. The younger child demonstrates more attachment behaviours, less easily modulated emotion, greater egocentricity, and magical thinking regarding malign events and distinguishing appearances from reality. Such metacognitive vulnerabilities in the young child are, therefore, seriously challenged in a situation where the mother is depressed, inattentive, unpredictable or delusional.

What is immediately apparent from this discussion on early developmental tasks is their inherent interdependence. It is difficult to speak of the child's social development apart from their cognitive or emotional development. Difficulty in one area clearly affects development in another. This is also true of the mother–child relationship.

Practitioners who are required to relate to each other in supporting the depressed mother and child may find themselves resorting to metaphors similar to those already employed by depressed mothers. Their expressions frequently reflect a relationship in need of attention, mutual understanding, reciprocity and good communication. Blocks to these interprofessional processes are comprehensively described by Woodhouse and Pengelly (1995) and may contribute to situations where the needs of depressed mothers and their children do not receive an adequate response.

Failing to meet the needs of the depressed mother and her child

Practitioners may find themselves dealing with a variety of behavioural and emotional problems in the child, for which mothers are seeking support, but which researchers have linked to maternal depression. Cummings and Davies (1994) address the complex issue of family-related processes and suggest that both parent and child characteristics will influence the developmental outcomes for the child.

Characteristics of age, gender and temperament are posited as important for a child's ability to manage the effects of the mother's depression. The effect of the mother's illness on the child may be ameliorated by internal and external factors, for example, the child's cognitive ability and personality, the presence of an adult in the family who is not ill, regular school attendance or making and keeping friends.

Extra-familial factors, such as socio-economic status, parental knowledge of child development, life stress and poverty, are also influential, mediating maternal depression and its impact on the child. However, it is also true that interaction among these various parent–child, familial and extra-familial factors can lead to neglect of the child, insecure attachment patterns and inappropriate maternal expectations of emotional and practical support from the child (Crittenden, 1992; George, 1996). Such psychological burdens may be borne by the child, but the consequences have been little researched (Radke-Yarrow et al., 1994; Zahn-Waxler, 1990).

Falkov's (1997) review for the UK Department of Health on child deaths makes it clear that some children are likely to be fatally harmed by their parents. He indicated that, of 100 reviews of child deaths, 32 showed evidence of parental psychiatric morbidity. Psychiatric morbidity includes severe forms of maternal depression and should, therefore, be a factor for consideration in child protection issues. This study indicated that nearly 40 per cent of ill parents had been in contact with mental health services before the child's death. The fact of having a mental health professional involved with severely depressed women should not, therefore, be seen as a protective factor in itself. What is most effective is recognizing that those parents who are most ill will not always have the ability to protect their own children from harm.

Attending to the needs of the depressed mother and young child is a daunting challenge to the single practitioner working in isolation. The depressed mother and child are in a dynamic system that is under stress. Clinicians and practitioners who do not work together experience similar stresses in their professional relationships. It is to this important issue that we now turn our attention.

Support from health professionals

Initial support for the depressed mother and her child is potentially available through the informal networks of family, friends and neighbours. Nevertheless, the nature of depression may damage these relationships, the mother's ability to access them and the willingness of others to help. Individual friendships, mother and toddler groups, playgroups, schools, primary health care providers such as midwives, health visitors and general practitioners, form the core community sources of support and initial contact for the depressed mother and child. These facilities are accessible without recourse to formal referral processes and are part of community life. Ostensibly, they function formally and informally and are user-driven. They are perceived differently, for example, from statutory social work or specialist medical intervention.

Women's experience of motherhood is most frequently observed and monitored in community settings, by health professionals, who make the greatest number of referrals to specialist resources such as paediatrics, community medicine, child and adolescent mental health services and social services.

Mothers most frequently express worries about early difficulties in establishing routine, managing and regulating emotions and managing behaviour to health visitors, general practitioners and in playgroups. However, it is often less obvious, in the early stages, to determine whether it is the child or the parent who needs help and such help may be difficult to obtain. Primary care staff, who attempt to access additional services for children and families, often discover that criteria for access to services differ within and between agencies and teams. If there are no clear indications of specific psychopathology in the child or the mother, likely imminent family breakdown or child protection issues, then any referrals they make are often not given priority by agencies such as social services or community mental health teams.

It is crucial that all professions have an understanding of the theory of child development so that they can make quality assessments and referrals to more specialist services when they are required. Integrated service provision, which is sufficiently flexible to intervene as soon as problems are identified, should be predicated upon the critical nature of the evolving relationship between mother and infant and its influence on the emotional well-being of the child. One in ten children and young people may have a mental health problem at any one time (Audit Commission, 1999). The availability of services, which recognize and deal with such problems early, could play a part in reducing child mental health problems. Implicit in this statement is the need to develop a relationship between individual practitioners, teams and agencies which will provide a positive model and continuity with the developing relationship between mother and child. In the UK, legislation is now in place which, in theory, can support such a model.

The Children Act 1989 defines a broad range of children for whom, and for whose families, services should be provided through inter-agency collaboration in both planning and providing services.

In, 1991, the UK formally accepted the recommendations of the UN Convention on the Rights of the Child, which incorporate the idea of a child with individual rights but in a dependent relationship with adults. This states in Article 19 that the state has an obligation not only to protect the child from all forms of maltreatment, but also to undertake preventive and treatment programmes relating to this.

Section 17 of Part III of the Children Act envisages that family support services should be offered 'to members of a family of a child in need where the service is provided with a view to safeguarding and promoting the child's welfare'. In assessing need:

> authorities must assess the existing strengths and skills of families concerned.... a chronically sick parent may need continuing practical and emotional support of varying degrees of intensity according to the incidence of acute phases of his illness and the developing needs of the child. (p. 6)

In this way, the law surrounding children's needs also requires a coordinated response from health professionals which support the related needs of other family members including the depressed mother.

Research on the views of practitioners working with the depressed mother and her child

In a study undertaken at the University of East Anglia, Gregory (1997) examined how a range of factors relating to the children of parents with mental health problems impinged upon the ability of professionals to make timely and appropriate responses to the assessed needs of those families.

Significant factors included: the profession of the referrer; the nature of the described problem; the thresholds for accessing services for mother and child; the quality of the working relationships between adult services and child care services; and whether the child or the parent was the subject of the referral for services. The degree of focus on the child as an integral part of a family system and the responses of different professionals to whole family situations were also examined. Semi-structured interviews were conducted with 22 mental health and child and family workers and the emerging themes were subjected to a grounded theory analysis (Glaser and Strauss, 1967).

Findings

The most significant professional issue emerging from the study was that 'situations' might be assessed but the individual needs of the child in the context of its family often went unacknowledged. This was in spite of the Children Act guidance which states that 'Careful joint assessment and planning are essential where families are vulnerable due to illness. Professionals whose primary concern is the mental health of adults should be fully aware that the welfare of any children should be evaluated in its own right' (p. 6).

Personnel in adult services were less likely to consider the child's individual needs if it was thought that further intervention, or a referral relating to the child's needs, would compromise the practitioner's relationship with the mother. One psychiatrist said: 'I do not always consider the needs of children – perhaps I should. The only time I do is when there are clear child protection issues.' In this study, only specialist children and families workers consistently assessed the individual needs of the child in the context of a whole family assessment. Others considered that legislation and local practice guidelines and procedures hindered a comprehensive assessment of the depressed mother and child, even when those specialist professionals identified a need.

The Health Advisory Service (1995) and the Audit Commission (1999) state that having a parent with a psychiatric illness increases a child's vulnerability to developing mental health problems in childhood. However, a child psychiatrist in Gregory's study indicated that sometimes the referrals he *did* receive were inappropriately directed, when the individual child may not have had a problem but was in a risky relationship:

> Not every child referred to me has a problem, but might be in a predicament. Referrers not infrequently ask for treatment in the absence of a problem.

A further emerging issue was the range of factors which mediated the ability of the workers to respond appropriately with a full range of services, and in a timely manner, to the needs of both the depressed mother and her child. One health visitor said:

> Because of high Social Services Department thresholds [criteria for providing services] I often feel as if I have to say the worst thing is happening in order to get a service.

Yet a social worker with children and families said:

> I am working with a mother who is very depressed and is emotionally unavailable to her children a lot of the time. She sees a Community Psychiatric Nurse once a fortnight but does not reach the threshold for services from a mental health social worker. I need to liaise closely with a mental health worker because I am not a mental health expert.

Paradoxically, if either child or parent is already receiving a specialist service, there can also be problems accessing other services because of inconsistent or inflexible service eligibility criteria. The assessments undertaken by workers who specialized in childcare related directly to their knowledge of the child's developmental needs relative to the capabilities of the parent. Even though all professionals said they were concerned about the effect on the child of the symptoms presented by the adult, individual practitioners and clinicians placed different emphases on the child's needs, relative to the parent's illness.

Overall, the study revealed significant gaps in knowledge about mental health as it affects mothers, child development as affected by parental mental illness, and the means of accessing services which would help both the mother and the child. Opportunities for consultation and joint working were neither well developed nor supported through intra- or inter-agency protocols.

Conclusion: towards coordinated and integrated preventive services

Mothers who suffer from depression do not have a full range of services available to them in the early stages of their illness. Falkov's (1995) and Glaser and Prior's (1997) studies demonstrate that some of their children are at risk of significant harm or death, if their needs are not recognized by professionals. However, the prevalence of maternal depression, its likely under-diagnosis (James, 1998) and the paucity of integrated, early, locally based and easily accessible services make it likely that the needs of some mothers and their children will not be met. Women whose depression is sub-clinical, misdiagnosed or undiagnosed are likely to become more isolated. Thus it is necessary for professionals to examine not only the phenomena of such depression and isolation but also the social forces, policies and institutional practices (including their own) which surround and shape these phenomena. (Hanmer and Statham, 1988).

Opportunities exist for professionals to support all parents who have a mental illness while also helping to protect children from the long-term effects of such illness. These opportunities exist not only in the high profile 'emergency responses', but also, and perhaps more significantly, in areas in which professionals have become less accustomed to working, in women's groups, in family support and in co-ordinated community responses to families in need. In respect of depressed mothers, the focus needs, additionally, to be one which explores and penetrates the broad social and economic contexts in which women must rear children.

Service planning for mothers and children needs to reflect the dilemmas faced by whole families, promote the support of both the mother's and the child's welfare, and provide a coordinated, integrated and accessible service. Recent legislation and guidance, described above, place an imperative on joint planning, provision of integrated services and interdisciplinarity which should have at their heart a focus on the needs of children in the context of their families. To this end, it is vital that practitioners, clinicians, trainers and policy-makers draw on the current recommendations in legislation and guidance in order to ensure that their services are coordinated and operate at a proper professional interface. This can be achieved through joint commissioning and service delivery models which support the role, function and relationships of professionals who, in turn, support the developing relationship between the depressed mother and her child. The nature of this support, however, can and should stretch beyond the exigencies of child protection, and a narrow definition of women as mothers and carers, to the well-being of these women in their own right.

Finally, as one author comments:

> To help the depressed mother and her family, it is necessary that we all keep up to date with new knowledge and that we add to that knowledge with our own ongoing research, projects and initiatives. All professionals must work together to achieve this end. (James, 1998: p. 167)

This brief review of theory and research has underlined the importance of using new knowledge to build effective and less fragmentary support for mothers with depression, by taking account of their wider familial and societal contexts, rather than acting on single factors in isolation.

Further reading

Cummings, E.M. and Davies, P.T., 'Maternal Depression and Child Development', *Journal of Child Psychology and Psychiatry*, 35 (1) (1994) 73–112.

Greig, A. and Howe, D., 'Social Understanding, Attachment Security of Pre-School Children and Maternal Mental Health', *Journal of Developmental Psychology*, 19 (2001) 381–93.

Kovacs, M. 'The Emmanuel Miller Memorial Lecture 1994. Depressive Disorders in Childhood: An Impressionistic Landscape', *Journal of Child Psychology and Psychiatry*, 38 (3) (1997) 287–98.

Murray, L., 'The Impact of Postnatal Depression on Infant Development', *Journal of Child Psychology*, 33 (1992) 543–61.

11

Can Women with Learning Disabilities Access Good Health Care? A Case Study of Cervical Screening

Christine Nightingale

Introduction

Women are frequent users of health services, not only for themselves, but also for those for whom they care – children, dependent adults and older people. Their ability to access good and appropriate health care, both in their own right and as caregivers is, therefore, of paramount importance (Pavalko, 2000). Some women are more skilled and able to access appropriate care. For example, individuals in higher socio-economic groups do better than those in lower socio-economic groups in accessing health care (Townsend and Davidson, 1988), and in their survival of cancer and heart disease (Phipps, 1999). Reasons for inequalities are many, ranging from communication skills through to affordability (Northam, 1996). Many studies of take-up of health care such as immunization, screening and health clinics, conclude that poor and less well-educated people are less likely to take up services, or to use them appropriately. This is a situation which is both costly and may contribute to some diseases re-establishing themselves in vulnerable and socially excluded groups without early interventions. There are indications of a continuing and 'growing division between the haves and have nots in our society' (Millman, 1993: p. 4).

In this chapter, I suggest that even established prevention services such as cervical screening are denied to some groups of women by a complex set of barriers. The chapter will explore both access and barriers to health care based on findings from a qualitative study on health access for women with learning disabilities which focused on cervical screening (Nightingale, 1997). The data show how these issues may affect whether many groups of women understand or are even offered the cervical screening service.

Cervical cancer

Cervical cancer occurs at the neck of the womb, where the vaginal canal and uterus meet. There are two forms of cervical cancer, adeno-carcinoma and squamous cell carcinoma. Adenocarcinoma is a rarer form, but it can occur in any woman whether she has been sexually active or not. The squamous variety accounts for 90 per cent of cervical cancers and is predominately linked with sexual activity, including early age of first sexual intercourse, number of sexual partners and after contracting sexually transmitted diseases, particularly vaginal warts or human papilloma virus (Grubb, 1986; Mihill, 1990; Singer and Yule, 1984).

In the United Kingdom, 2,000 women die each year from cervical cancer. Of these, 88 are thought to be preventable deaths had the cancer or pre-cancerous signs been detected earlier by screening (Smith and Jackson, 1988). Pre-cancerous changes to the cervix can be successfully treated, halting the progression of the condition. Detection by cervical screening is a relatively simple procedure undertaken in most general practice surgeries, family planning and Well Woman Clinics, saving the lives of 800–1,000 women annually (Boseley, 1999). The smear test, which involves scraping a sample of endo-cervical cells from the cervix with a cervical spatula or brush, is usually painless, though many women may experience discomfort and embarrassment. As Harris notes (Chapter 1, this volume), it is an invasive and personal procedure, and gives rise to concerns from the screeners themselves (Nightingale, 1997), yet such discomfort is rarely acknowledged even within the health education and promotion literature.

Learning disability

Women with learning disabilities are as eligible for screening as other women. However, they have a label which is broad, confusing and easily misunderstood. Some may have severe learning disabilities, leaving them with poor receptive and expressive communication as well as poor cognitive processes, while others live independent lives. Some will have been sexually active, either by choice or through abuse

(Brown, 1992); others will not. It is important to be clear that labelling a woman as having a 'learning disability' does not necessarily indicate low levels of communication, poor understanding or lack of sexual experience. None the less, this label creates a barrier for some primary health care practitioners.

Women with learning disabilities are often, though not always, socially excluded, and unable to manage in social structures because of their lack of social capital. They may have few contacts, limited education and employment skills, and lack contact with support and education agencies.

Research on women and cervical screening

Literature

Research on UK cervical screening for women with learning disabilities started in 1989. During the 1980s, there had been increasing research interest in cervical cancer and screening services, investigating causation, treatment, screening call and recall rates. Although none of this specifically addressed the needs of women with learning disabilities, some of it explored other disadvantaged or excluded groups of women in inner-city areas (Celentano et al., 1989), in social classes IV and V (Koopmanschap et al., 1990), and from other cultures, particularly Asian women (Havelock et al., 1988b). Some women from specified research populations were noted as being excluded from screening, with indications that these might be seen as more 'difficult to manage'. These might be women at risk but with psychiatric and psychological problems (Ross, 1989) or 'other conditions' (Havelock et al., 1988a). One study by a general practitioner followed up women who had not responded to their cervical screening invitation. He reported that he had excluded 'those few who were likely to respond unfavourably, such as a Mongol and a schizophrenic patient' (Plaut, 1986: p. 47). Other studies that investigated non-attendance among women to their cervical screening invitation often concentrated on ways of encouraging non-attenders into health programmes by sustained attempts at contact (Beardow et al., 1989; Elkind et al., 1989; Pierce et al., 1989).

Most of these studies were based on service concerns, such as achieving a high take-up of cervical screening. One study, in contrast, considered the woman's needs, and examined attitudes, knowledge and experience of cervical screening of women in Tower Hamlets

(Savage et al., 1989). Of 635 women who were interviewed, only 11 per cent understood the purpose of cervical smear tests, and women with the least education were least likely to have had a smear or to have understood its purpose.

Since the 1980s, few studies have examined rates of cervical screening attendance. Media interest has focused on laboratory errors leading to false results and poor health outcomes for the women concerned (Boseley, 1999; Quinn, 1999). There has, however, been an increased interest in the quality of service provision for people with learning disabilities including, specifically, cervical screening (Djuretic et al., 1999; Hall and Ward, 1999; Pearson et al., 1998; Stein and Allen, 1999; Whitmore, 1999). This interest is currently generated mostly from specialist practitioners and researchers who work with people with learning disabilities rather than from generalist researchers or general practitioners.

Research context and method

The qualitative research described herein was prompted by three personal experiences. First, was the death, from cervical cancer, of a woman with severe learning disabilities who had never had cervical screening. Second, was the difficulty of persuading one woman with gynaecological symptoms even to consider seeing her doctor about something unrelated to her learning disability and epilepsy. Third, was the reluctance of many family practitioner (GP) teams to include women with learning disabilities in their women's health screening programme.

Consequently, the research focused on whether women with learning disabilities were offered cervical screening and the ways in which this service was afforded or denied them, in order to examine how far this group of women had equality of access. Conducted in a large, mainly rural, health authority, it explored the mechanisms and processes of the cervical screening service from the perspectives of those staff most directly involved in health care delivery – those working in general practice. All 78 general practice partnerships in one health authority were invited to participate; 62 took part and a total of 140 interviews were conducted with the general practitioners, practice nurses and practice managers. All interviews with general practice staff were individual, semi-structured and explorative and took place in the general practices. No researcher definitions about learning disability, access or cervical screening were offered, so that constructs were developed by the respondents.

Table 11.1   Interpretation of Reading Ease Score

Score	Level of difficulty	Per cent who would understand	Typical magazine	IQ required for comprehension
0–30	Very difficult	4	Scientific	126 + (superior)
31–50	Difficult	24	Academic	111 + (bright normal)
51–60	Fairly difficult	40	Quality	104 + (bright average)
61–70	Standard	75	Digests	90 + (low average)
71–80	Fairly easy	80	Slick fiction	87 + (dull normal)
81–90	Easy	86	Pulp fiction	84 + (dull normal)
91–100	Very easy	90	Comics	81 + (dull normal)

Source: Adapted from Ley (1973: 8).

Both general practices' letters of invitation for cervical screening and their cervical screening health promotion leaflets were analysed in detail for their readability, presentation, message content and, where applicable, pictures. Standard tests were used to measure the accessibility of texts (Ley, 1973). This involved identifying:

- a score derived from a word and syllable count;
- matching the score to identify a reading level or identified 'reading age';
- the IQ required to comprehend the text;
- the percentage of the population who would be able to understand the text (see Table 11.1).

Tests were also used to measure 'Human Interest' (Flesch, 1949), based on how familiar the text is and whether it addresses the reader directly by using words like 'you' or 'your'. The level of interest is obviously critical in health promotion, for engaging readers and encouraging them to take an appropriate health action.

Five women with learning disabilities, who met at a women's group, also took part in the research process. They agreed to arrange a group meeting with me to discuss cervical screening. As this group arranged its own agenda, usually around health issues, its members were untypical of many other women with learning disabilities living in the same research area who were often isolated, had communication difficulties and low levels of social capital. However, they were typical in that two of the five women lived at home with relatives, two were in a group home and one lived independently.

Access and barriers to health care

Access is probably most easily measured when there is a clear course of action for a known condition. Millman (1993: p. 5) defines access as 'the timely use of personal health services to achieve the best possible health outcomes'. This study demonstrated that barriers to health care were complex and rooted in every aspect of health administration and practice through: ineffective policy; inadequate communication and information; lack of understanding; and decisions made which exclude patients themselves. These are described in the sections below.

Policy

Cervical screening developed from small, nationally-run initiatives (DHSS, 1981a; 1981b) through to a massive operation delegated to regions and local management by health authorities. The National Health Service aim is relatively simple. According to the Department of Health guidelines, all women between the ages of 20 and 64 are eligible for cervical screening (DHSS, 1988). No national policy documentation suggests by explicit exclusions that any particular group of women should be denied access to screening.

Department of Health correspondence confirms that women with physical or mental disabilities should not only be included, but that hospital managers should pay special attention to such women:

> I must stress that all women within health authorities, regardless of physical or mental disability, if aged 20–64 years will be included in the current screening programme. Hospitals for either disability should ensure their patients are included in the programme. (Department of Health, 1992, personal communication)

Nevertheless, the regional or health authority level interpretation of central government policy produced potential grounds for excluding various groups of women. Local health service guidelines issued at that time to general practitioners in one health authority listed some groups of women who could be 'cancelled' from cervical screening programmes as:

- women with total hysterectomies;
- *mentally subnormal patients* [my emphasis];
- the medically inappropriate (terminal illness, or those for whom a smear is impossible to perform, for example, a woman with rheumatoid arthritis);

- those with a sex change;
- patients who have never been sexually active (this *may* include female members of the church). [my emphasis]

A number of access issues emerge here in terminology and decision-making. First, the UK Department of Health had not used the term 'mentally subnormal' for more than a decade prior to this statement being written and its terminology was being changed to 'learning disability' as these local guidelines were being published. This suggested that the originators of the guidelines clearly had little recent professional knowledge of the women they were writing about. Additionally, the terminology applied to each category of 'cancelled' or excluded women, suggests some difficulty in coming to terms with all those listed being acknowleged as women. The only category that acknowledges their gender is that of 'women with total hysterectomies'. Women with learning disabilities and celibate women were described as gender-less 'patients'. Men or women who have had a 'sex change' are referred to as 'those', again genderless. Finally, these guidelines offer no suggestion that the decision to cancel screening should be undertaken with informed consent from the women themselves.

Policies developed by the general practices researched in the study were also explored. None of the general practices interviewed had a written policy or guidelines for the administration and management of cervical screening. Cervical screening services were organized within the cultural norms of each practice giving rise to individual practices managing women's access to cervical screening in a variety of ways. The names of women due for a cervical smear were sent from the health authority to each general practice. Letters inviting women for cervical screening were sent out either from individual practices or, centrally, from the health authority. Either way, the general practice staff would check the lists of women's names sent to them and confirm their eligibility. Criteria for eligibility included administrative details about whether they were alive, at the same address and still registered with that particular general practice. However, the interviews also revealed that more subjective judgements were made about the individual women, and were drawn on to generate an extensive list of reasons for 'cancelling' women from screening (see Table 11.2).

The list of reasons given for not calling in a woman for screening could be divided into three groups: objective reasons, generalized reasons and emotional reasons. First, objective reasons, could be seen to be reasonable and practical, as with pregnancy, hysterectomy and

Table 11.2 Reasons, given by general practices, for temporary removal of women from cervical screening

Item (in the words used by interviewees)	Items mentioned by different practices
'Hysterectomy'	46
'Pregnancy'	10
'Under treatment for other diseases'	4
'Mental handicap'/'Subnormal'/ 'Mongol'	10
'Virgins'	7
'Professional virgins' (nuns)	5
'Physical disability'	4
'Illness'	3
'Emotional disorder'	1
'Trauma'	2
'Upset by smear'	1
'Currently not sexually active'	2
'Personal knowledge'/'experience (of the patient)'	3
'General health'	2
'General doubts about the woman'	2
'Spinsters'	2
'Parkinson's disease'	1
'Psychiatric disorder'	1
'Terminal illness'	3
'Previous abnormal smear'	2
Total number of mentions	**111**

Source: Nightingale (2000).

terminal illness. Second, generalized terms such as physical disability, psychiatric and emotional disorder and women who have experienced trauma, may well result in excluding or 'cancelling' women who may well be concerned to ensure that their cervix is healthy. Third, are terms which carry an emotive charge: 'virgins'; those with 'emotional disorder'; 'trauma'; those 'not sexually active' and 'spinsters'. There is little evidence that general practitioners were fully aware of the sex life of all the women in their practices. Few would know if women were virgins, and assumptions were made about unmarried women (spinsters) and nuns. Few women would be able to say that they had never fallen into one of the potential cancellation categories at some stage of their lives.

Department of Health policy (1988) was reasonably inclusive as far as women with learning disabilities were concerned. This study demonstrated, however, that further down the implementation chain, barriers to access for screening could be erected without women ever knowing that they were excluded.

Communication and information

Women with learning disabilities often have poor communication skills and levels of social capital with which to attempt to obtain ordinary health care entitlements. Only in one general practice did a mechanism exist for recording any communication difficulties, but even this one lacked a procedure for assessing or following up such communication problems. An invitation to attend general practices usually relied on the written word. Letters were sent out to all women. If they did not respond, two or three more letters were sent. After that, their notes were marked so that opportunistic contact could be made, for example, when the woman next presented herself for a health appointment.

Despite reports (ALBSU, 1987) of increasing levels of illiteracy among the population, none of the general practices had developed procedures to allow for variable levels of reading. During the interviews, practice staff acknowledged that they simply had not considered what might happen if a woman were unable to understand their letters:

> I have to say we are not aware of illiteracy in the practice, I think you are raising our consciousness. (General Practitioner 16)

> They wouldn't be able to read the letter, would they? – oh yes that's a problem, you might think they were non-responders, wouldn't you? (Practice Nurse 28)

> I don't know who can't read. If there was a parent or other member of the family group – hopefully, doctors would be more aware – I haven't thought about that. (Practice Nurse 34)

The assumption made by practice staff was that:

> Most people have access to readers. (Practice Nurse 51)

> One would assume that someone else was reading for them. (General Practitioner 23)

This might be 'someone else in the household' (General Practitioner 9), 'people' generally (General Practitioners 18, 14, 23, 40), and 'the man' [husband or partner of the woman who couldn't read] (General Practitioner 39). Others, however, assumed that those patients who could not read were incompetent in all aspects of their lives and in need of care and support:

> If they cannot read, they cannot do anything in society. (General Practitioner 33)

> No, don't know of anyone who can't read. The whole family has to be incapable of reading [for it to be a problem?] ... If they live on their own they wouldn't stand an earthly. (Practice Manager 58)

Women were invited for cervical screening by letter. Besides notifying women that they were due for the test, some of these letters would briefly outline the need for the test, some enclosing information leaflets produced by pharmaceutical companies and charitable organizations.

Through the study, thirteen cervical cancer or cervical screening leaflets were identified in the health authority and two further leaflets were obtained direct from the publisher. The quality of the leaflets and the depth and accuracy of the information in them was variable, sometimes compounding the confusion of the letters.

The content of the leaflets were analysed using the Flesch (1949) and Ley (1973) formulae, described above, varying considerably in their readability scores. The best had a score of 80.3, 'very easy', judged to be readable by a majority of the reading population and with a 'very interesting' Human Interest Score. At the other end of the scale was a leaflet which scored 56.3, 'fairly difficult', requiring a level of reading competence at an academic book level, with a 'dull' Human Interest Score. There was no evidence of a quality control process of critical selection of leaflets to determine how far they met the needs either of the general practices, or of their patients with whom they needed to communicate.

While beliefs expressed within the leaflets were not necessarily those held by the practice staff, women might assume the practice had validated the beliefs by sending the leaflet to them. For instance, some leaflets expressed the view that women who had not been sexually active were not at risk of developing cervical cancer:

> Cervical cancer is connected in some way with sexual intercourse and is not found in virgins. (Health Education Authority, 1988)

While these women may have been at low risk, they might still be at risk from other cancer-causing factors. As mentioned already, in 10 per cent of cases, adenocarcinoma can occur whether a woman has been sexually active or not. Such information creates a barrier by conveying a false belief that a sexually inactive woman is not at risk from cervical cancer.

Understanding

It has been suggested earlier that women should be given the opportunity to make a choice about whether to have cervical screening or not. Central to women's ability to choose and gain access to health services must be whether they first receive, and understand, information about cervical cancer and screening.

Within the study, a commonly encountered assumption of both general practitioners and practice nurses was that women patients knew what the cervical screening procedure was about. In the interviews, none of the practice staff said that they regularly described or explained cervical screening to women. When pressed, some practice nurses said that, if asked, they would verbally describe the procedure to patients, or resort to hand-drawn diagrams at the time of the consultation. Cervical screening is hard to describe, especially as it requires an understanding of the internal arrangement of vagina, cervix and uterus. Because of this difficulty, it was clear that many practitioners actually tended to avoid explaining it, even when it was badly needed by particular patients. Without that information, women may not be able to give informed consent, and may experience an invasive examination, which might be interpreted as an assault.

Study interviews with a group of five women with learning disabilities revealed that two of them had little or no idea of what cervical screening was or what it was for. Another two had undergone smear testing, having quite different experiences, but in both cases with a very limited understanding of why they had had a smear. This was illustrated by one of the women (Ms D), who asked for information but was refused in a patronizing way. Ms D has a good understanding of what is said to her. A slight speech impediment and a slowness of speech hamper her verbal skills, but nevertheless, she is articulate and clear:

Christine: Were you prepared? Did you have enough information?
Ms D: No.
Christine: So, when you went in and actually had it done [cervical smear], did anyone say what they were looking for and what they were going to do?

Ms D: No, but I did ask.
Christine: You did ask?
Ms D: I did ask, but they didn't tell me.
Christine: What did they say when you asked?
Ms D: I was not to talk about those things, it would worry me.

This led Ms D into an unpleasant and distressing experience, which could be described as assault, given that she had no adequate information and, therefore, no informed consent.

Christine: So, what was the smear test like?
Ms D: It was bad.
Christine: Bad?
Ms D: Yes, I didn't like it.
Christine: What didn't you like?
Ms D: It hurt, was uncomfortable, they didn't tell me, no.

Decisions by others

The final factor to be discussed here is the barrier created by removing health decision-making from a woman with learning disability. It was assumed by most of the general practice staff interviewed that no woman with a learning disability was competent to make a decision or give consent. Practice staff often transferred the power of decision-making to non-medically trained people, such as parents and carers. For example, one practice manager said that 'parents had said that the smear was not appropriate' (Practice Manager 29). Some general practices suggested that they 'decided with relatives' (General Practice 38) and would 'contact the family or helper or minder' (Practice Nurse 17). However, there was evidence that not all parents were listened to, especially if their views ran contrary to those of the practice staff team. A community nurse told the story of a mother who believed her daughter should have cervical screening but the general practitioner thought it unnecessary and refused. Few health practitioners echoed the beliefs of one general practitioner who felt that he should not be making unscientific judgements about women:

I would hate not to send for women who would actually respond to invitations because you were erroneous in your perceptions of whether they would come or not. (General Practitioner 39)

Leaving the individual out of the decision-making process is entirely against any advocacy or empowerment principle (Williamson, 1993). Clearly, some women with the most severe learning disabilities will find such participation very difficult. Here a good advocate must be found who can intelligently weigh up the benefits and the harm of asking a woman who has limited understanding to take part in a very invasive procedure. Ross (1989) argues that making decisions on behalf of patients is the art rather than the science of medicine. It is clear that such 'art' may be helpful, but can be detrimental to individual needs and ability to self-determine, especially where it is based on personal prejudice or the evidence of a third person.

Conclusion

This chapter has highlighted some of the barriers that exist for women with learning disabilities in accessing cervical screening. Cervical cancer is a detectable disease, which can occur in any woman with a cervix regardless of her current or previous levels of sexual activity. The test for cervical cancer and pre-cancerous signs is relatively simple, but it is invasive. It may also be interpreted as abusive if there are any doubts about whether the woman has given informed consent. Previous research (Savage et al., 1989) has shown that many women, not only those with learning disabilities, do not understand the purpose of cervical screening, which means they cannot give informed consent. Unfortunately, the present research showed that many health practitioners did little to explain cervical screening. Many relied on the health promotion literature, some of which contained misleading information. Health practitioners need to examine the basis of the health communication and advice that they offer to patients and ensure that they agree with its content and accuracy.

National screening policy in the UK (DHSS, 1988) shows that all women within certain age limits are eligible for screening, yet local policy and the limiting practice of health practitioners can place restrictions, often unseen, on access to care. A woman with learning disabilities, like other women deemed by local health practitioners to be unsuitable for screening, may be unaware that her name has been removed from the call-up list.

Furthermore, little account was taken of individual communication needs, particularly of women who have poor literacy. All invitations for screening in this study were sent out by letter, with poor follow-up for women who did not respond and make a screening appointment.

Where the form of communication was inappropriate for some women, this created a barrier to their health care access. Health providers should make themselves more aware of their patients' communication needs and explore alternative means of making contact – for example, telephone or personal visit.

Barriers to health care were found at all stages and levels of the health provision service, from policy, through the administrative process, to face-to-face delivery. Providers should systematically evaluate their services through the policy trail from national policy to the point of delivery. Using a case study to examine the service from the perspective of the most vulnerable women enables the evaluator to focus on specific needs such as physical access, cultural matters, literacy and other communication issues.

The case of women with learning disabilities highlights how women who are vulnerable because of their disability, health status, cultural and language differences are at risk from barriers to health care which exist because their specific needs have been ignored.

Further reading

Hall, P., Ward, E., 'Cervical screening for women with learning disability: Numbers screened can be optimised by using a focussed initiative', *British Medical Journal,* 318 (1999) 536–37.

Nightingale, C., 'Barriers to health access; a study of cervical screening for women with learning disabilities', *Clinical Psychology Forum,* 137 (March 2000) 26–30.

Pavalko, E.K. and Woodbury, S., 'Social roles as process: caregiving careers and women's health', *Journal of Health and Social Behaviour,* 41 (1) (2000) 91–105.

Salganicoff, A. and Wyn, R. 'Access to care for low-income women: the impact of Medicaid', *Journal of Health Care for the Poor and Underserved,* 10 (4) (1999) 453–67.

Part IV
Building Health in Policy and Practice

12
Health Policy and Provision for Maternity Care in the United Kingdom in the Twentieth Century

Miranda Mugford and Alison Macfarlane

Introduction

Examining changes in maternity care policy can help demonstrate how women bring about real changes in their own and their families' health care. Over the twentieth century, public provision of maternity services in the United Kingdom was driven by a combination of policy influences, particularly by concerns about mortality in children and women. The result has been a highly centralized, medicalized and 'technological' service for pregnancy and childbirth care. However, since the 1970s, women campaigners, health care professionals and researchers have highlighted the need for services to take fuller account of the role of women in decision-making, both about their own lives and in public life (Garcia et al., 1990; Oakley, 1981). In England, the government's *Changing Childbirth* initiative (Department of Health, 1993) raised the possibility that maternity care might be provided differently in the future.

This chapter examines trends in and reasons for provision of various aspects of maternity care, and then considers the role that women can take and have taken in shaping maternity services. It is written by an economist (MM) and a statistician (AM), both women, with a professional interest in the evidence about maternity health care policy. Our main focus here documents trends in birth and maternity care in England and Wales, linking them to changes in the focus of national policy. This series of developments has often been analysed individually in socio-political terms, but we will review the impact of political and economic pressures on the development of maternity care in Britain.

174   *Miranda Mugford and Alison Macfarlane*

Trends in births, care and outcomes

Current patterns of maternity care are the result of a long process of development and change, which can be described using government statistics. Elsewhere, we have described and presented these sources of data in some detail (Macfarlane and Mugford, 1984; 2000; Macfarlane et al., 2000). Here we give some examples of what they tell us about births, their outcomes and the context in which they occurred during the twentieth century.

Many of the statistics are collected as the by-product of legal or administrative processes. Birth and death registration date back to the mid-nineteenth century and were established primarily for legal purposes. As the state commenced to fund maternity services and then to provide them, statistical systems were set up to monitor, first, the services provided and, later, the care received by individual women and babies.

Births and mortality in the twentieth century

The general fertility rate in England and Wales has fallen over the last hundred years. Thus fewer babies are born per thousand women of childbearing age, as Figure 12.1 shows.

Figure 12.1   General fertility rate, England and Wales, 1838–2000

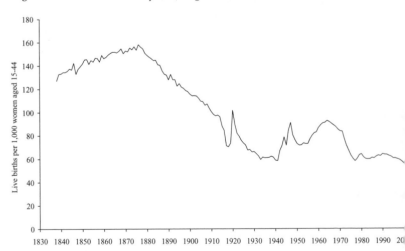

Similar trends occurred in other countries of the United Kingdom with fertility rates remaining highest in Northern Ireland. Women are also much less likely to die around the time of childbearing now than 150 years ago, when about six women died per thousand babies born alive in England and Wales. Just under five did so in the 1930s. The rate then plummeted to one death per thousand births by 1950 and to below one per ten thousand in the 1980s and 1990s (Macfarlane and Mugford, 2000). Babies are now much more likely to be born alive and to survive the first year of life. In 1846, the infant mortality rate in England and Wales was 163.5 per thousand registered live births. The rate fell from 154.2 in 1900 to 29.9 in 1950 and 5.6 in 2000, as Figure 12.2 shows.

The overall fall in mortality in the twentieth century has not, however, been steady and continuous. When rates fluctuated, this provoked public, professional and political reactions. These then affected aspects of policy, public spending and health care. Thus, there was concern about infant mortality in the early years of the twentieth century, about maternal mortality in the 1930s and about perinatal mortality in the late 1970s.

Figure 12.2 Infant mortality, England and Wales, 1846–2000

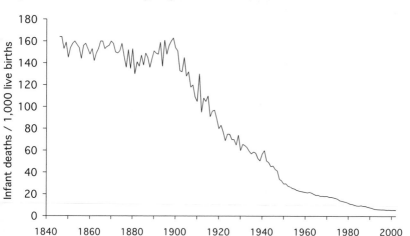

Trends in overall mortality rates can mask what happens in particular sub-groups. For example, in the early twentieth century, the biggest reductions in infant mortality occurred in the post-neonatal period, that is, among babies aged at least one month but under twelve months. Rates of neonatal death, that is, deaths of babies under 28 days of age, dropped less dramatically at this period, but decreased steadily throughout the twentieth century.

Babies at the highest risk of dying are those born with low birthweight and/or before term. The lower their weight and gestational age at birth, the greater is their chance of dying. Mortality rates tend to vary both geographically, and between social classes. This is partly a consequence of differences in factors such as the incidence of low birthweight. Figure 12.3 shows that babies with fathers in unskilled manual occupations in Registrar General's social class V are more likely to be of low birthweight than those with fathers in professional occupations in Registrar General's social classes I or II. The proportion of low weight births is even higher among babies whose birth is registered solely by their mother.

Low birthweight is also much more common among multiple births than among singleton births. There has been poor recognition of the additional needs for health and social care arising from multiple birth, however (Botting, Macfarlane and Price, 1990). As in many other developed countries, the proportion of multiple births rose during the 1980s and 1990s in England and Wales, after many years of decline, as Figure 12.4 shows. The increase was particularly marked among triplet and higher order births.

These trends may be partly due to mothers' increasing age at childbirth, as multiple births are more common among older women. Yet multiple birth rates are rising in all age groups, except among women aged under 20. This suggests that the rise is a consequence of the increasing availability and use of techniques for the medical management of sub-fertility.

The social context of birth changed in many ways during the twentieth century. Fertility rates and average family sizes fell with the increasing availability of contraception. Family structures changed, with increasing numbers of births outside marriage and rising rates of divorce, lone parenthood and remarriage. There were parallel changes in women's roles and patterns of paid employment.

The relationships between poor family circumstances, infant mortality and low birthweight are well documented and are reflected in the persistent social class differences shown in Figure 12.3. The numbers of

Figure 12.3 Low birthweight by social class of father, births within marriage and jointly registered births outside marriage, England and Wales, 1999

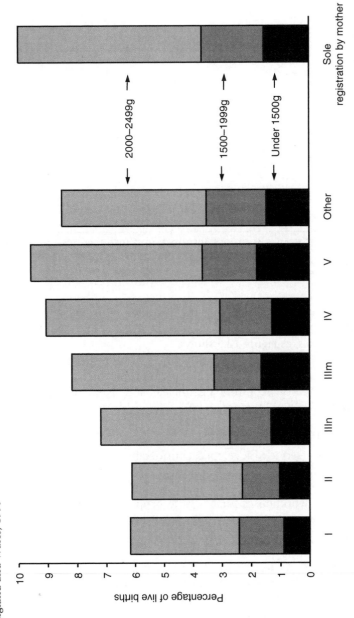

Source: Office for National Statistics, Mortality statistics, Series DH3

Figure 12.4   Multiple birth rates, England and Wales, 1938–2000

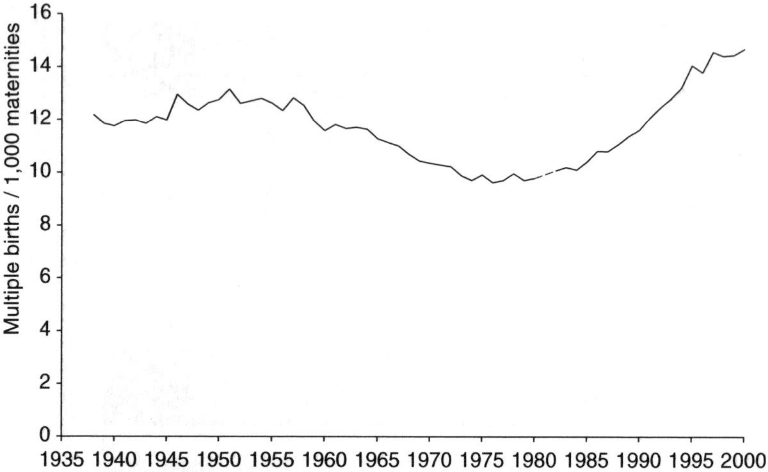

Source: Office for National Statistics, Birth statistics, Series FM1
Graph by Alison Macfarlane, City University

people in households on low incomes with children, increased between 1961 and 1993, as part of a general widening in social inequalities, as Figure 12.5 shows.

Paradoxically, social class differences in stillbirth and infant mortality rates did not widen over the period from the late 1970s onwards, but the reasons for this are unclear and need further exploration (Macfarlane and Mugford, 2000).

Maternity services and care

Maternity services developed considerably over the first half of the twentieth century. At the beginning of the twentieth century, just over 1 per cent of deliveries took place in institutions, either the 'lying-in' wards of workhouses for destitute people, or charitable institutions specifically providing maternity care. Everyone else gave birth at home. Maternity homes for women without complications, and specialist obstetric units in voluntary hospitals and workhouse infirmaries, were established in the 1920s and 1930s (Campbell and Macfarlane, 1994). By 1946, 53.7 per cent of births took place in institutions (Joint Committee of RCOG and PIC, 1948). After the National Health Service began in 1948, the demand for hospital maternity care grew and facilities were developed. The percentage of home births in England and

Figure 12.5 Individuals in households with children below half average income, before housying costs, Great Briitain, 1961–93

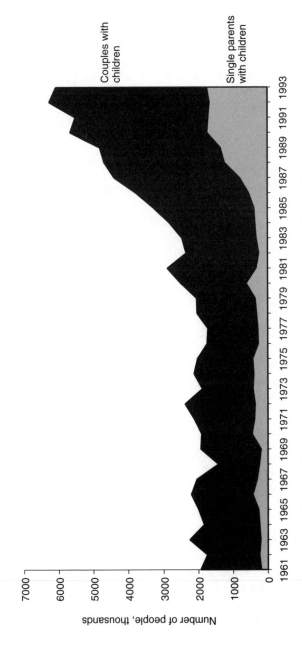
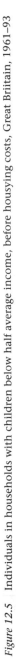

Couples with children

Single parents with children

Number of people, thousands

7000
6000
5000
4000
3000
2000
1000
0

1961 1963 1965 1967 1969 1971 1973 1975 1977 1979 1981 1983 1985 1987 1989 1991 1993

Source: Analysis of Office for National Statistics Family Expenditure Survey data by the Institute for Fiscal Studies

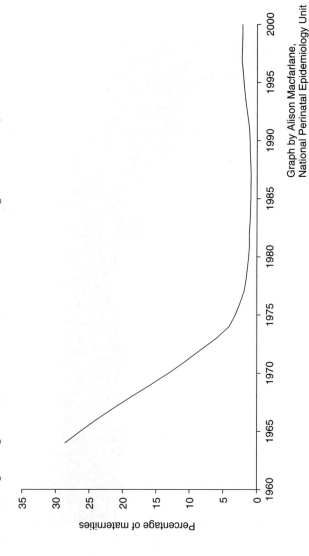

Figure 12.6 Percentage of registered maternities which occurred at home England and Wales, 1964–2000

Source: Office for National Statistics, Birth statistics, Series FM1

Graph by Alison Macfarlane,
National Perinatal Epidemiology Unit

Wales declined rapidly in the late 1960s and early 1970s, as Figure 12.6 shows. By 1987, only 0.9 per cent of deliveries in England and Wales took place at home. Changing views in the late 1980s led to a small but steady rise, with about 2.2 per cent of deliveries taking place at home at the end of the 1990s (Campbell and Macfarlane, 1994; Macfarlane and Mugford, 2000).

The rising numbers of births in hospital have increasingly been concentrated in ever-larger units with fewer beds in smaller units, and closures of many community maternity units. These changes have been accompanied by the development of facilities for neonatal intensive care, usually located in the larger hospitals (Macfarlane and Mugford, 2000). In 1996, nearly a quarter of births in the United Kingdom were recorded as taking place in units, with 4,000 or more births in that year (Macfarlane and Mugford, 2000). As Figure 12.7 shows, under 3 per cent of births in 1996 took place in units with fewer than 1,000 births.

As Savage has noted (Chapter 7), it was not until the early 1990s, following the publication of *Maternity Services* (House of Commons Health Committee, 1991) and *Changing Childbirth* (Department of Health, 1993), that women's right to informed choice about place and nature of childbirth, and midwives' overall responsibility for many women with uncomplicated pregnancies giving birth in hospital settings, came to be formally acknowledged.

In parallel with the trend towards hospital delivery, the use of medical intervention has increased. Caesarean sections are increasingly used for delivery as Figure 12.8 shows. It is difficult to interpret recent trends, as the statistical data for England and Wales were interrupted by a change in health information systems during the 1980s.

Examples from maternity policy: some stories behind the statistics

Public provision of maternity care in the UK has evolved with the wider health services. The service has moved from care provided by local authorities and independent practitioners, for people who were eligible or could pay, to a service where everyone registered with the NHS can have midwifery care, primary health care, secondary level obstetric and paediatric services and, if needed, referral to tertiary specialist services.

In this section we relate the trends just described to three interrelated strands in policy and development of services for pregnant women and their babies. These are policies for mothers' and children's

Figure 12.7   Total births by size of maternity unit, United Kingdom, 1996

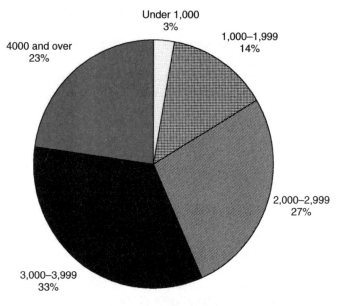

Source: Macfaclane A., Mugford M. *Birth counts: statistics of pregnancy and childbirth*, Tables A7.1.1–A7.1.4

Births by size of maternity unit, 1996

	England	Wales	Scotland	Northern Ireland	
All units	604705	33300	57,717	24,163	719885
Less than 10	162	4	0	0	166
10–199	4438	727	1553	40	6758
Under 200	4600	731	1553	40	6924
200–999	10341	515	1015	2102	13973
1,000–1,999	66489	9948	12204	9254	97895
2,000–2,999	157470	14587	11370	9727	193154
3,000–3,999	215855	7519	17140	3040	243554
4,000 and over	149950	0	14435	0	164385

All units	719885
Less than 10	166
10–199	6758
Under 200	6924
200–999	13973
Under 1,000	20897
1,000–1,999	97895
2,000–2,999	193154
3,000–3,999	243554
4,000 and over	164385

183

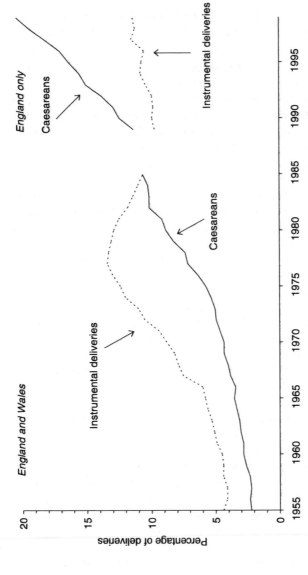

Figure 12.8 Operative delivery rates, 1955 to 1999/2000

Source: Ministry of Health, Department of Health and Social Security, Welsh Office, Office of Population Censuses and Surveys, *Maternity Hospital In-patient Enquiry* and Department of Health, *Hospital Episode Statistics*.

health, the place of delivery and the costs of childbearing for families and society. Where possible, we illustrate points at which women may have influenced the changes in maternity provision.

'Woman-centred' care – from neonatal mortality to women's satisfaction: a tale of House of Commons committees

Children's and mothers' mortality and health were already issues of concern to nineteenth-century social campaigners. Public and government interest in the population's health was stimulated by the poor health of potential recruits to the Army for the Boer War at the beginning of the twentieth century. In response, some local authorities set up services such as 'milk depots' or 'schools for mothers' for pregnant women or those with young children. The working-class Women's Co-operative Guild campaigned for antenatal, delivery and child health services, and health insurance to cover health costs of childbirth (Llewellyn Davies, 1915). In 1919, a Ministry of Health was established with one of its four main aims being 'to secure the health and welfare of childbearing women and infants'. This was the responsibility of its maternal and child welfare department, headed by Janet Campbell, with a staff of women doctors, nurses and midwives (Ministry of Health, 1920).

Maternal mortality was investigated in reports and enquiries by Campbell and other Ministry of Health staff (Campbell and Macfarlane, 1994; Macfarlane and Mugford, 2000) Although infant mortality was falling, maternal mortality increased slightly during the 1920s and early 1930s, before dropping sharply from the mid-1930s onwards. The Registrar General's Decennial Supplement showed, unusually, that in the early 1930s wives of professional men had higher maternal mortality rates than wives of men in unskilled occupations (General Register Office, 1938). This may partly be explained by the greater opportunity for middle- and upper-class women to have a doctor to attend their birth, or to deliver in a nursing home, exposing them to greater risks of operative intervention and/or infection (Donnison, 1977; Loudon, 2000). In one 'experiment' in Rochdale, campaigns to inform women and health care practitioners of the dangers of obstetric intervention were encouraged by the Medical Officer of Health. They were followed by a decline in maternal deaths (Oxley et al., 1935).

After a substantial fall in maternal death rates by the 1950s, public attention turned again to babies. Perinatal mortality rates, that is rates of stillbirth and death in the first week of life, were not falling as fast as death rates among older babies. Successive official enquiries led to medical and public pressure for more NHS facilities for neonatal care for ill newborn babies and also for monitoring pregnancy and labour more intensively (Committee on Child Health Services, 1976; House of Commons Social Services Committee, 1980) This pressure coincided with the development of technologies for electronic fetal monitoring and for life support in very small babies. It led to calls that every maternity unit should have minimum standards of provision for monitoring, resuscitation and intensive neonatal care. Public campaigns for the expansion of neonatal care claimed it would eliminate disabilities such as cerebral palsy. These campaigns, involving women who had experienced loss or preterm birth, proved successful. During the 1980s, facilities were expanded so that, by the end of the twentieth century, it had become the norm for very preterm babies, born at very low weights and gestations, to have intensive neonatal care. In response to this, in 1992, the birth registration laws in the United Kingdom were amended to lower the limit for registration of fetal deaths as stillbirths from 28 to 24 completed weeks of gestation.

This rapid expansion of neonatal care was achieved at the cost of 'normal' maternity care. The high cost of equipping and staffing a neonatal unit, together with the relatively small numbers requiring such care, brought considerable pressure to centralize services, with many obstetric units merged so that births would occur close to neonatal units. Although numbers of medical staff involved in neonatal care grew during the 1980s, nurses were in short supply. Many midwives moved into specialist neonatal care, reducing ratios of midwifery staff to births in hospital maternity care.

These changes gave rise to increasing dissatisfaction about the quality of experience for women giving birth in hospitals (Garcia et al., 1990; House of Commons Health Committee, 1991). Rates of maternal and infant mortality had now fallen so low that the 'safety' issues were dwarfed by the questions of whether women were healthy, could feed their babies, and were reasonably content, capable parents. Despite this shift in policy, surprisingly few data are available to monitor most of these outcomes at national level (Audit Commission, 1997).

Hospital or home birth – women's choices and 'health resource efficiency'

When the NHS began, women were guaranteed access to free health care and midwifery services, but not to a hospital delivery. Concerns that specialist maternity care was being denied some women who needed it led to the formation of a campaign group, the Association for the Improvement of the Maternity Services (AIMS). The organization still campaigns for appropriate use of technology, but is more active in campaigning against inappropriate intervention and for home births. A major hospital building programme in the 1960s and 1970s led to a large increase in numbers of obstetric beds. By the 1970s, the postwar baby-boom had passed and the birth rate declined. As a result the demand for hospital birth could be met, and it was felt that some maternity hospital beds were being underused. In 1970, a report by the Standing Maternity and Midwifery Advisory Committee stated that:

> We think that sufficient facilities should be provided to allow for 100 per cent hospital delivery. The greater safety of hospital for mother and child justifies this objective. (Standing Maternity and Midwifery Advisory Committee, 1970)

Although no evidence was given to support this statement, subsequent reports repeated it and general practitioners in primary care became increasingly nervous of their medical responsibilities for births. These two influences alone might explain the sharp fall in home births from 1965 onwards shown in Figure 12.6.

In fact, a review of the relevant research concluded that there was no evidence for the claim that the safest policy was for all women to give birth in hospital, nor for the policy of closing small obstetric units on the grounds of safety (Campbell and Macfarlane, 1987). It also suggested that home delivery and use of midwifery-led units would cost less than centralized obstetric hospital care for both the NHS and women themselves (Campbell and Macfarlane, 1994; Henderson and Mugford, 1997). Groups representing women, providers of community-based maternity care and women politicians such as Audrey Wise participating in the parliamentary enquiry into maternity services, used such research for campaigns to widen choice over place of delivery.

In England and Wales, the percentage of births at home had started to rise from the late 1980s, as Figure 12.6 shows. This signalled a change of mood and moves towards midwife-led care, reflected in policy documents and initiatives across the UK and following on from the Select Committee reports discussed earlier.

Changes in household economics, reproductive technologies, and the case of multiple births

The economic circumstances in which births occur were a central concern throughout the twentieth century. Before the NHS, the cost of maternity care was a major worry for women. Successful campaigns, first for national insurance coverage for childbirth and, later, for the NHS to provide free maternity care, made a considerable difference for poor families especially those where medical difficulties occurred. There are also wider costs of child-bearing for women and families, including the obvious costs of caring for a baby, and the less obvious cost of giving up earnings or other activities (Joshi et al., 1999).

In Figure 12.5, we show trends from the 1960s to the early 1990s in numbers of people in low-income households with children, with child poverty and single parenthood becoming increasingly common. These data reflect economic trends of increasing income inequality during the last two decades of the twentieth century, and changing patterns of marriage, childbearing, and working. These changes have affected parents' needs for support of children and for care during and after pregnancy and childbirth.

Provision of state support for families has lagged behind social changes. For example, until 1987, payments of maternity benefit were made only to women who had paid qualifying insurance contributions. Unemployed, temporary and part-time workers were not entitled, yet were probably most in need of the extra support. The work of the Maternity Alliance increased public awareness of this inequity, deliberately echoing the much earlier campaign of the Women's Co-operative Guild (Gowdridge, 1997). Changes in the 1990s provided a somewhat more generous and inclusive benefit scheme.

Debate about the role of the family, the benefits and disadvantages of women's paid employment inside or outside the home and whether they have had equal opportunities at work has been highly polarized. It has been set against the overall trend during the twentieth century, of more child-bearing women participating in the workforce. The increase in women's earning potential has meant a corresponding increase in foregone potential earnings as a result of pregnancy, maternity and child-rearing (Callender et al., 1997; Joshi et al., 1999).

The changing patterns of workforce participation and costs of childbearing, coupled with the opportunity to choose when to have a baby, may partially explain the trends in fertility discussed above. Figure 12.4 also shows a rapidly increasing rate of multiple birth in the last two decades. A national survey of triplet and higher order births in the early 1980s found that there was clearly a considerable extra cost burden associated with these births (Botting, Macfarlane and Price, 1990) compared with a singleton baby. Parents of triplets were involved in planning the research, and the Twins and Multiple Births Association used the results in campaigning for better health and social services and welfare benefits. Since this survey, changes in recommended clinical policies for management of fertility treatment have been adopted and the use of assisted conception has expanded. However, an additional maternity benefit allowance for parents with high order births was not granted.

What role for women in defining maternity services and policy in future?

This inevitably partial history none the less illustrates several factors in the development of maternity services and support for parents. There are clearly many ways in which women have influenced events since the earliest years of the twentieth century. We can also see the contribution of demographic, technological, cultural and economic change in defining the importance of specific issues at particular times.

Women had a role in all of these wider social changes to the extent that they were able to influence decisions about work, fertility, and family formation. They also influenced specific changes in maternity policy, whether as service recipients, as campaigners or as providers or commissioners of care. It is easy to point to examples of paternalistic decisions, such as schemes of antenatal care and the move towards increased intervention and larger hospitals. It is also possible to find examples where women were closely involved in influential decisions, or policy development about maternity care. They included civil servants, such as Janet Campbell in the 1920s and others in the 1990s, health care staff and managers, members of women's organisations and individual women politicians.

Campaigning groups have always been active in maternity care, playing many different roles. At the beginning of the twentieth century, the Women's Co-operative Guild campaigned for clinics, delivery and home visiting services. In the inter-war years, the National Birthday Trust Fund, an organization of upper-class women, campaigned on maternity issues. In the postwar era, it provided the funding base for a series of national surveys of births and the conditions in which they occurred (Williams, 1997) The Association for Improvements in the Maternity Services (AIMS) was founded in the 1960s, alongside the National Childbirth Trust (NCT). The Maternity Alliance was formed in 1980 specifically to campaign about rights and benefits, while many other organisations represent specific client groups such as parents with multiple births, or raise funds for particular aspects of care, such as equipment for neonatal units. These groups have had influence by reporting on current experiences of maternity and neonatal care, by lobbying, media campaigning and fundraising, and by providing evidence to official investigations and being represented on local and national advisory bodies.

There have been developments in the formal structures for public consultation and decisions in the NHS, and for including lay views in decisions. In maternity care, following the 1980 report by the parliamentary Social Services Committee (House of Commons, 1980), maternity services liaison committees were set up in every district to provide a forum for medical, midwifery, primary care and lay representatives to discuss local maternity services. Successive changes in health service organization have altered how decisions are made about where to provide services and what to provide. Since 1999, local health services are commissioned by primary care groups or trusts, with committees comprising mainly general practitioners to represent local primary care providers in purchasing secondary care, including maternity services, for people in their catchment populations. These groups have usually one lay member to represent the very wide range of lay concerns about health care provision, not just those of women and babies. Although 'woman-centred' and 'midwife-led' care have become common terms in the organization of maternity care, the choices on offer to pregnant women in any local setting are restricted by longer-term decisions already made about health service provision. Although pregnant women have some choice in the clinical care they receive, and are probably more informed than in the 1970s and 1980s, a longer view is needed to ensure their needs are considered in decisions about service development.

In all of the examples given in this chapter, there is a common theme concerning the role of belief and the power of evidence. In the case of the place of delivery debate, and the expansion and central-ization of labour ward technology and neonatal care, services were developed on the basis of guidance from doctors' organizations, but largely in the absence of unbiased research evidence about what is effective.

From 1989 onwards, the publication of the Oxford Database of Perinatal Trials, and its successor, the Cochrane Library, provided a strong base of regularly updated evidence about the effectiveness of alternative forms of care (Chalmers, Enkin and Keirse, 1989; Cochrane Collaboration, 2000) taken from systematic review of randomized trials. These, in turn, have been dominated by drug or technology studies, not always addressing other important questions, notably about service users' views and experiences. An increase in midwife-led and user-led research in maternity care is beginning to fill some of the gaps, however (Oliver, 1999).

Another aspect of evidence, important in the development of maternity care, is the availability of information about what is happening, and how it is experienced. Our description of events has been based on national official statistics, which cover a limited range of issues, excluding areas such as postnatal health or satisfaction with services. As a result, information to monitor changes in such policy areas is available only through specially organized research.

We have been able to give only a few specific examples of the very wide range of issues and policies, which both involve and affect women in maternity care. This means that we have not presented data about the involvement of women as health workers, a clear 'emerging theme', considered in depth elsewhere (Donnison, 1977; Garcia et al., 1990). We have also concentrated on evidence about UK maternity services. Much more can be learned from the different experiences of the ways in which maternity care has evolved in other countries (Declercq, 1998; Declercq and Viisainen, 2000).

Our analysis of the development of maternity care during the twentieth century suggests that those involved in provision and reform in maternity care have based their campaigns on different sources of evidence, within the context of changing economic forces. Evidence from national statistics and narrowly focused research, particularly about mortality risks, has been used in support of political and medical policies. On the other hand, the experiences of individual women have been the basis for campaigns to relieve poverty and improve the experience of childbirth. We have illustrated that conflicts have arisen where groups relied on different sources or interpretations of evidence. Each source has strengths and gaps. Increasingly, public and clinical policy makers are encouraged to incorporate evidence about the views of users of services while some representatives of users' interests are making use of statistical evidence and are involved in evaluative research. Such a merging of approaches implies an interdisciplinary approach to both campaigning and policy-making.

However far this is taken, there will always be conflicts of wishes and values between different groups making and affected by any policy, in the face of limited resources. Women are clearly affected by maternity policy, but are also involved in making policy. They may attach varying weight to particular types of evidence or policies, and may exert their influence through campaigning and other political activities, membership of clinical professions, or management of the health service. As we have shown, women were actively involved in all these ways throughout the twentieth century, and are likely to take a more central role in the twenty-first century.

Acknowledgement

Alison Macfarlane was funded by the Department of Health at the time this chapter was written.

Further reading

Campbell, R. and Macfarlane, A., *Where to be Born? The Debate and the Evidence*, 2nd edn (Oxford: NPEU, 1994).

Garcia, J., Kilpatrick, R. and Richards, M., *The Politics of Maternity Care: Services for Childbearing Women in Twentieth-century Britain* (Oxford: Oxford University Press, 1990).

Macfarlane, A. and Mugford, M., *Birth Counts: Statistics of Pregnancy and Childbirth* Volume 1 Text, 2nd edn (London: The Stationery Office, 2000).

Macfarlane, A., Mugford, M., Henderson, J., Furtado, A., Stevens, J. and Dunn, A., *Birth Counts: Statistics of Pregnancy and Childbirth*, Volume 2 Tables, 2nd edn (London: The Stationery Office, 2000).

13
Ethnicity and Inequalities in Older Women's Health

Helen Cooper and Sara Arber

Introduction

The neglect of social inequalities in older people's health has been fuelled by implicit assumptions that old age brings universal ill-health and that health promotion strategies for older age groups will meet with only limited success (Ginn et al., 1997). The emergence of an 'ageing society', with a growing proportion of the population over working age, challenges these assumptions. Projection of current UK trends suggests that, by 2016, the number of adults aged 65 and above will exceed those under 16 years (Office for National Statistics, 2000). The percentage of women over 65 years increased from 14 per cent in 1961 to 18 per cent in 1998. The equivalent figures for men are 9 per cent and 13 per cent, demonstrating the predominance of women in later life. This chapter uses survey data to explore how the social characteristics of older people in Britain, in terms of gender, ethnicity and socio-economic circumstances, are related to health outcomes at age 50 to 74 years.

The current living circumstances and socio-economic position of older women and men contribute to inequalities in health and health-related behaviour; low occupational class, poor material circumstances, living alone or being widowed are all associated with adverse health outcomes. These disadvantaged groups include a disproportionate number of older women, due to gender differences in occupational class and employment history, as well as life expectancy.

Although socio-economic circumstances are recognized as important determinants of older women's health, many large-scale studies on older women can be accused of being 'ethnocentric'. The health of older minority ethnic women is rarely investigated and little is known about how socio-economic position may differentially affect the health of white and minority ethnic women at this stage of life. Large-scale British surveys show that different ethnic groups vary markedly in their access to a range of socio-economic and material resources, with Pakistani and Bangladeshi adults more likely to occupy positions of low socio-economic status than any other ethnic group (Nazroo, 1997). However, we do not know the contribution of socio-economic position to gender differences in morbidity within ethnic groups or to ethnic differences in health among women.

The 'invisibility' of older minority ethnic women in UK health research is partly because minority ethnic adults – and women in particular – form a very small proportion of the older population. In 1998–9, only 9 per cent of Black Caribbean adults and 7 per cent of Indians in the UK were above retirement age (65 years) compared to 16 per cent of whites, and for Pakistanis and Bangladeshis the figure was much lower at 3 per cent (Office for National Statistics, 2000).

The neglect of health issues for this group is compounded by their assumed 'cultural difference' from the white majority – for example, that their health needs will be catered for within supportive family networks, or, that they will 'return to their homeland' in later life (Ahmad and Walker, 1997; Blakemore and Boneham, 1994). It is important to investigate the relationships between gender, age, ethnicity and health as the number of older minority ethnic adults, and their use of health and welfare services, will dramatically increase over the next two decades (Ebrahim, 1996).

Among the current generation of older minority ethnic adults – the vast majority born outside the UK – women have had a very different life-course from men, tending to migrate later and at an older age (Blakemore and Boneham, 1994). The employment participation of women varies by ethnic group, with much lower levels of paid employment among women from the Asian subcontinent than for white or African-Caribbean women. We need to know, therefore, how gender combines with ethnic group and socio-economic resources to influence the reported health of older minority ethnic women.

Age, gender and ethnic inequalities in health

Theories of jeopardy

Researchers in America have claimed that minority ethnic adults experience 'double jeopardy' in old age, with the combined disadvantages of age and racial discrimination. This has been linked to greater health inequality between older black and white Americans (Dowd and Bengston, 1978). The economic and social barriers associated with old age and a minority ethnic status are viewed as doubly detrimental to older people's health and provide an explanation for the high levels of morbidity among older black Americans. Other authors have extended theories of jeopardy to incorporate additional inequality associated with inequitable access to health services (Norman, 1985) or gender (Palmore and Manton, 1973). We use the term 'triple jeopardy' in this chapter to refer to the threefold disadvantages that may be experienced by older minority ethnic women; age, race and gender discrimination.

These theories of 'jeopardy' are, however, contested. While socio-economic disadvantage and discrimination are considered to have undoubted negative consequences for health, some have argued that ethnic differences are not exacerbated in later life. Rather, ethnic differences in health may be a persistent feature of the life-course. Or else, old age may transcend ethnic boundaries, reducing socio-economic or health inequality across ethnic groups (Kent, 1971). This argument implies that old age 'levels out' ethnic inequalities in health, and greater social support or the revered status of older people from minority ethnic groups is often cited as an advantage. The 'triple health burden' associated with being an older minority ethnic woman has also been criticized because jeopardy assumes that ethnic, gender and age inequality have cumulative effects on health, rather than these factors 'intersecting together to produce specific effects' (Anthias and Yuval-Davis, 1992: p. 100).

Socio-economic inequality and health

In Britain, there has been little systematic investigation of the disadvantages that may be experienced by older minority groups and how these may be structured by gender. Large-scale British surveys have drawn attention to the high morbidity of many minority ethnic adults aged 16 or above, based on self-reported measures of general health and chronic illness (Nazroo, 1997). These studies have shown that ethnic inequalities in health are closely related to the degree of socio-economic disadvantage experienced by minority ethnic groups, with the greatest ill-health among the most materially deprived Bangladeshi group. Current knowledge about ethnicity and health in old age is largely based on small-scale surveys or qualitative work in one locality, often focusing on the health of one ethnic group, such as 'Asian'. However, these studies do suggest that older minority ethnic adults –

particularly women – experience multiple social disadvantages which impact on health. Employment during working life largely determines economic and material resources in old age, through access to benefits, pensions and savings for example. In the UK, more women than men have low income in later life because of their interrupted employment histories associated with child-rearing, higher levels of part-time work and gender disparity in earnings (Ginn and Arber, 1999).

There are also marked differences in labour force participation figures within ethnic groups. Pakistani and Bangladeshi women have much lower levels of economic activity than Black Caribbean and white women. This may reflect norms and expectations about the role of women in domestic work, child-care and paid employment (West and Pilgrim, 1995), but official figures are likely to obscure the high level of unregistered or 'home-based' work undertaken by Asian women, with low pay, status and long work hours. A study of older Asians living in Bradford (Ahmad and Walker, 1997) reported that very low literacy and fluency in English was an additional barrier that often prevented these women from securing welfare benefits, including state pensions, cold-weather payments and free bus passes.

Overall, there is evidence that minority ethnic women are discriminated against in terms of pay, promotion prospects and job status compared to white women (Patel, 1993), probably increasing the dependence of older minority ethnic women on other family members or means-tested benefits. Thus, it can be seen that greater material hardship and economic insecurity, coupled with added difficulties in accessing health and social services, are likely to contribute to ethnic inequalities in older women's health.

Behavioural differences and health

While some researchers emphasize high levels of socio-economic disadvantage among minority ethnic women, others focus on 'cultural differences' between ethnic groups as explanations for health inequalities. The concept of 'culture' is often reduced to an essentialist notion of 'lifestyle' and many studies have suggested that explanations for ethnic inequalities in health can be found in the health-related behaviour of minority ethnic groups. These arguments have often underpinned health promotion targeted at minority populations; examples include efforts to reduce the incidence of rickets by changing 'Asian' diet and living habits (Rocheron, 1988). From this perspective, culturally-based health beliefs and norms are believed to structure individual behaviour and thus influence health status.

However, the argument that ethnic differences in health are mediated by culturally determined behavioural choices has been contested. It is argued that an undue focus on culture neglects material explanations for ethnic differences in health and often serves only to 'pathologize' cultures and 'blame the victim' for poor health (Ahmad, 1993). The concept of culture is often applied to minority ethnic groups in a mechanistic way, implying a stable and fixed set of 'rules' that deviate from the 'norm' of the white majority. The diversity of culture within ethnic groups (including white groups), and similarities across cultures, are often neglected when 'ethnic group' and 'culture' are used interchangeably.

Aims and methods

This chapter analyses two British national surveys of black and Asian communities, commissioned by the Health Education Authority (HEA) in 1992 and 1994 (HEA, 1994; 1999). To permit comparison across ethnic groups, this is supplemented with data for white adults from an HEA of Health and Lifestyles conducted in 1992 (HEA, 1995). We focus on the 50–74 age group because of an upper age limit of 74 years in these surveys. We investigate how theories of jeopardy, socio-economic disadvantage and health behaviour relate to ethnic inequalities in the reported health of older women aged 50–74.

The relationships between ethnicity and age are firstly examined to assess whether arguments of jeopardy may be relevant in a British context. Our results would be consistent with arguments of 'double jeopardy' if older age and a minority ethnic status is associated with the greatest ill-health. To assess whether older minority ethnic women face a threefold health disadvantage (or 'triple jeopardy') associated with old age, gender and ethnicity, we present separate results for men and women in each ethnic group.

We then examine whether ethnic inequalities in older women's health can be attributed to differences in the socio-economic character-istics of minority ethnic and white women, based on measures of occu-pational social class and material resources. Finally, we analyse a key aspect of health-related behaviour. We focus on the tobacco consump-tion of older women from different ethnic groups, using information about current cigarette smoking and the practice of chewing tobacco by older Asian women. From our results, we assess the likely contribu-tion of 'cultural differences' in smoking behaviour and socio-economic disadvantage to ethnic inequalities in older women's health.

Data used in the analysis

The Health Education Authority (HEA) conducted surveys in 1992 and 1994 of Black and Minority Ethnic Groups (BMEG) (HEA 1994, 1999), which contain a larger sample of older minority ethnic adults than is available in most other nationally representative surveys. These BMEG surveys include information about self-reported health, cigarette smoking and tobacco chewing, as well as the socio-economic characteristics of men and women. Self-reports of health status and health behaviour are commonly used in social surveys, but we acknowledge that lay perceptions of 'good health' may vary for different ethnic groups in old age.

The 1992 BMEG survey interviewed 3,550 and the 1994 BMEG survey interviewed 4,452 adults from black and Asian communities (HEA, 1994; 1999). For both years, sample selection was based on Census Enumeration Districts (EDs) where 10 per cent or more of the population lived in households where the head of household was born outside the UK, according to the 1981 Census (HEA, 1994).

As the BMEG surveys focus exclusively on minority ethnic groups, comparable information has been analysed for white adults from the 1992 Health and Lifestyles Survey (HALS) conducted by the HEA (HEA, 1995) which interviewed 1,395 older white people aged 50–74 and is similar in design to the BMEG surveys. However, the HALS is based on a nationally representative sample of the UK, whereas only areas of high minority ethnic concentration were sampled in the BMEG surveys. Both the BMEG and HALS surveys selected one eligible respondent from each household. Our analysis focuses on the 1,561 women and 1,630 men aged between 50 and 74 in the combined BMEG and HALS data-set.

Gender and ethnic inequality in older people's health

Our analysis of health inequality among older age groups is based on a commonly used global measure of ill-health, namely self-assessed health. This is measured in the HEA surveys by the question 'Compared to others of the same age, would you say your health is very good, fairly good, fairly poor or very poor?'

Figure 13.1 compares ethnic inequality in health for men and women aged 16–49 with older age groups of adults aged 50–59 and 60–74. All four minority ethnic groups were more likely than white adults to report poor health and this was more evident for Asian

198 *Helen Cooper and Sara Arber*

Figure 13.1 Percentage reporting 'fairly poor' or 'very poor' general health by ethnic group and age
[*Base numbers in brackets*]

Adults aged 16–49

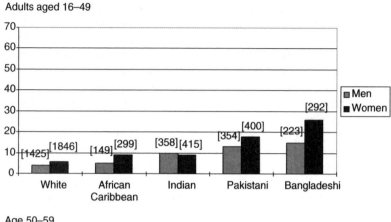

Age 50–59

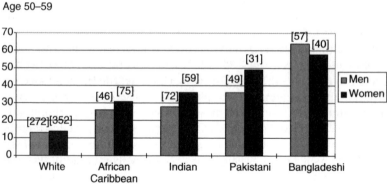

Age 60–74

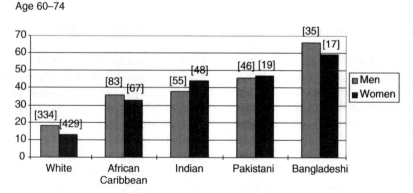

Source: HEA HALS (1992) and HEA BMEG (1992 and 1994)

groups than for African-Caribbean adults. Whereas approximately 5 per cent of white adults aged 16–49 reported poor health, this increased to 15 per cent of Bangladeshi men and 27 per cent of Bangladeshi women. Pakistani and African-Caribbean women were also more likely than men in these groups to assess their health as poor.

The health disadvantage of minority ethnic groups was most marked for adults aged 50–74 (see Figure 13.1), where more than half of Bangladeshis reported 'fairly poor' or 'very poor' health compared to under 20 per cent of older whites. The proportion of older African-Caribbean, Indian and Pakistani adults rating their health as poor was also substantially higher than for the white majority. Our analysis of age, ethnicity and health showed ethnic inequalities in health were amplified in older age groups, but were not unique to this stage of the life-course (Cooper et al., 2000).

African-Caribbean, Indian and Pakistani women aged 50–59 appeared more likely to report poor health than men in their fifties from these ethnic groups, whereas there was no gender difference in health for white adults in their fifties. However, a health disadvantage was not evident for older Bangladeshi women and reported ill-health was only greater for Indian women than for men in the 60–74 age group. Overall, our results do not suggest that older minority ethnic women are in a position of 'triple jeopardy' for poor health. The most striking finding is of ethnic inequalities in general health which become more marked in older age groups, rather than gender inequalities in reported health.

However, our assessment of jeopardy theories is limited by the use of cross-sectional survey data in this study. Differences between age groups could be partially influenced by age-related factors such as cohort effects, historical period and migration (Blakemore and Boneham, 1994). A more adequate assessment of jeopardy would therefore require longitudinal data showing ethnic and gender differences in health for the *same* individuals as they age.

Socio-economic disadvantage and ethnic inequalities in women's health

Older minority ethnic women are much more likely than white women to report poor health. We now examine how these ethnic inequalities in health are related to the socio-economic position of older women. Using measures of occupational social class to capture the socio-economic position of older people is sometimes considered problematic because information about previous occupation must be used for those who have left the labour market many years earlier. None the less, social class gradients in reported health have been found for older men and women based on their current or previous occupation (Arber and Cooper, 1999).

For older women, and a sizeable proportion of older Asian women in particular, there are additional problems about how to classify women not previously in paid employment. However, these difficulties do not negate the importance of connecting socio-economic circumstances to the health of men and women from minority ethnic groups.

Figure 13.2 examines social class inequalities in the reported health of older white and minority ethnic women based on their current or last main occupation. The question on class in the 1992 BMEG and HALS surveys excluded the long-term unemployed (more than six months), sick or disabled and those looking after the home, but retired adults were asked about their last main occupation (HEA, 1994; 1995). We present a separate category for women 'excluded' from the class measure, since this accounts for the majority of older Asian women.

Despite the limitations of the social class measure, Figure 13.2 shows social class gradients with a higher proportion of white, African-Caribbean and Indian women aged 50–74 in the manual social class

Figure 13.2 Percentage reporting 'fairly poor' or 'very poor' general health by ethnic group and Registrar General's social class: women aged 50–74 *[Base numbers in brackets]*

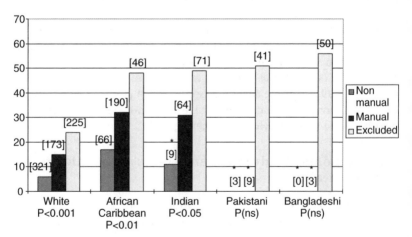

* Denotes base number less than 10

Source: HEA HALS (1992) and HEA BMEG (1992 and 1994)

reporting poor health. Over 30 per cent of African-Caribbean and Indian manual women reported morbidity which was halved for African-Caribbean women in the non-manual social class. Reported poor health among older white women was 15 per cent for the manual social class and only 5 per cent for those classified in non-manual occupations.

Very few older Pakistani and Bangladeshi women were allocated a class position, thus highlighting the limited ability of this social class measure to represent the socio-economic position of these women. For each ethnic group, reported morbidity was greatest for older women who were excluded from the class measure. For white and African-Caribbean older women in particular, health status may determine economic activity, with poor health necessitating an early exit from the labour market. However, this is unlikely to be the case for older Pakistani and Bangladeshi women who have a very low level of economic activity.

The relative contribution of social class and other socio-economic variables to ethnic inequality in older women's health is examined using logistic regression in Figure 13.3. The first bar represents the odds ratios (OR) of reporting 'fairly poor' or 'very poor' general health for

Figure 13.3   Odds ratios of 'fairly poor' or 'very poor' general health by ethnic group: Women aged 50–74

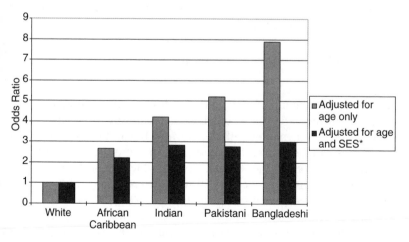

*includes social class, highest educational qualification, housing tenure and car availability

Source: HEA HALS (1992) and HEA BMEG (1992 and 1994)

women from different ethnic groups after adjusting for variation associated with age (measured in 5-year age groups).

The second bar shows how these ethnic differences are modified by controlling for a range of socio-economic factors. Substantially higher odds ratios of poor health were found for all minority ethnic women; the odds ratios were over five times higher for Pakistani women and more than seven times higher for Bangladeshi women, compared to the reference category of white women (OR 1.00), demonstrating marked ethnic inequalities in health for older women.

When the analysis was adjusted for structural characteristics based not only on women's social class but also their educational level, housing tenure and car availability (Figure 13.3), the health disadvantage of minority ethnic older women relative to older white women was greatly reduced. This strongly suggests that socio-economic disadvantage makes a large contribution to ethnic inequalities in older women's health. It does not, however, fully account for the high morbidity reported by minority ethnic older women as significant ethnic variation in health is still evident in Figure 13.3. For example, the odds ratios of poor health for older Bangladeshi, Pakistani and Indian women remain approximately three times higher than for older white women. In part, this may reflect the limited ability of existing socio-economic measures to represent the social status of older minority ethnic women. However, it could also be suggested that there may be an alternative explanation, which centres on 'cultural differences' in health behaviour, and this is discussed in the next section.

Smoking behaviour of older white and minority ethnic women

To assess the argument that cultural differences in 'lifestyle' may underlie ethnic variation in older women's health, we focus on one health behaviour, namely differences in tobacco consumption. Our analysis is based on current cigarette smoking and the use of chewing tobacco among older Asian women, both of which are health-damaging. Figure 13.4 examines gender and ethnic differences in current cigarette smoking for older women and men aged 50–59 and 60–74.

Current cigarette smoking for white men and women in their fifties was comparable at just over 30 per cent, but women were markedly less likely to smoke cigarettes in all minority ethnic groups. Only a small proportion of minority ethnic women in their fifties were smokers; this was true of less than 10 per cent of African-Caribbean and Pakistani

Figure 13.4 Percentage currently smoking cigarettes by ethnic group and age [*Base numbers in brackets*]

Age 50–59

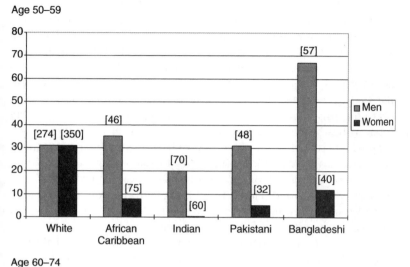

Age 60–74

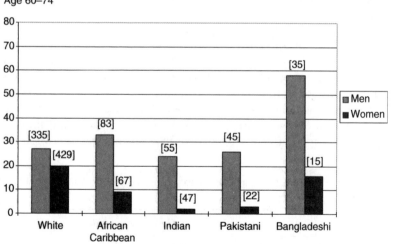

Source: HEA HALS (1992) and HEA BMEG (1992 and 1994)

women, approximately 12 per cent of Bangladeshi women and only 1 per cent of Indian women. In contrast, reported cigarette smoking was comparable to that of white men for African-Caribbean and Pakistani men, and smoking among Bangladeshi men far exceeded that of white men at nearly 70 per cent.

In the 60–74 age group there was a similar pattern of very low smoking among minority ethnic women compared to men in these groups. White women over 60 were less likely to smoke than white men, but smoking was still more commonly reported by white women than minority ethnic women; less than 5 per cent of Indian and Pakistani women were smokers compared with 20 per cent of white women.

As well as measures of cigarette smoking, the BMEG surveys asked about the use of 'smokeless tobacco' by Indian, Pakistani and Bangladeshi women. This refers to the practice of adding tobacco to an oral chewing mixture referred to as 'betel-quid' or *paan*. Chewing tobacco has been linked with the development of oral cancers, and even when tobacco is not added to the chewing mixture, it may still be carcinogenic (Bedi, 1996). Our measure of tobacco chewing is based on whether older Asian women reported that they chewed betel and tobacco and/or used *paan*. Combining information on reported cigarette smoking and tobacco chewing, Table 13.1 shows the overall tobacco consumption of older Asian women.

The table confirms that over 80 per cent of Indian and Pakistani older women did not smoke cigarettes or use chewing tobacco. However, a greater proportion of women from these ethnic groups reported chewing tobacco than smoking cigarettes. No Indian or Pakistani women combined cigarette smoking and tobacco chewing. In marked contrast, only 7 per cent of older Bangladeshi women did not report smoking cigarettes and/or chewing tobacco. Tobacco use was largely confined to tobacco chewing alone among 78 per cent of older Bangladeshi women. However, some 12 per cent of Bangladeshi women aged 50–74 reported that they chewed tobacco *and* smoked cigarettes. The health consequences of tobacco-chewing have yet to be

Table 13.1   Cigarette smoking and tobacco chewing* among Asian women aged 50–74

	Indian	Pakistani	Bangladeshi
No use of cigarettes or tobacco	85	92	7
Chew tobacco only	14	5	78
Smoke cigarettes only	1	3	2
Smoke cigarettes and chew tobacco	0	0	12
%	100%	100%	100%
N=	221	102	116

* Defined as use of betel + tobacco and/or the use of *paan*.
Source: HEA BMEG (1992 and 1994).

systematically explored for UK minority ethnic populations, but oral cancer and pre-cancerous lesions are reportedly more common in India for adults who chew tobacco (Bedi, 1996).

Discussion and conclusions

There were substantial ethnic inequalities in reported health among older adults, aged 50–74 years, and our results suggested that the health disadvantage of minority ethnic groups was more marked among older adults than for younger adults. The associations between ethnicity, age and health provide some support for 'double jeopardy' theories of health inequalities; namely that older minority ethnic adults must contend with a double burden of age and race discrimination on health. However, there was less evidence in our analysis that patterns of poor health among older minority ethnic women could be characterised as 'triple jeopardy'. Within older minority ethnic groups, reported poor health was not consistently greater for women than for men. However, longitudinal survey data are needed to examine how the relationships between age, ethnic group and gender change over time for the same individuals. As the older minority ethnic population increases over the next few decades, the differential effects of ageing on white and minority ethnic women and men will assume greater significance in health research.

A much greater proportion of older minority ethnic women reported poor general health than older white women. This was most evident for Pakistani and Bangladeshi women, especially health-disadvantaged by their socio-economic position. The likelihood of reporting poor health was significantly related to the class position of older African-Caribbean and Indian women, and the health disadvantage of all minority ethnic women was greatly reduced after controlling for socio-economic differences between white and minority older women.

While the importance of socio-economic factors for older women's health was affirmed, our study found no evidence that cigarette smoking among minority ethnic women could be an explanation for ethnic differences in health. A striking finding was the very low level of cigarette smoking among all minority women aged 50–74, particularly older Asian women. Among older women, it is paradoxical that the best health is reported by the ethnic group with the highest level of smoking, namely white women. If ethnic inequalities in health were mediated by cigarette smoking, one would expect to find the greatest morbidity among older white women.

There was a marked difference in the use of chewing tobacco by older Asian women. Chewing tobacco was more prevalent among Indian and Pakistani women than cigarette smoking and the majority of older Bangladeshi women reported chewing tobacco. It would, however, be misleading to conclude that chewing tobacco is a wholly cultural practice causally related to the high level of poor health reported by older Asian women. To understand this behaviour, we need to contextualize tobacco chewing in the broader framework of these women's lives. A main criticism of cultural explanations, as applied to studies of ethnic difference, is that culture is not a static phenomenon, but may be shaped by social factors including gender, socio-economic circumstances and previous life experiences (Ahmad, 1996). Just as cigarette smoking among older women is highly correlated with low socio-economic position and a lack of material resources (Cooper et al., 1999), so tobacco chewing may be related to wider social circumstances that constrain or promote this behaviour. The potential influence of socio-economic circumstances on health may therefore be mediated by patterns of health behaviour.

Better health for all older women and men requires that we tackle the disadvantaged socio-economic circumstances which are closely associated with poor health. Many older people from minority ethnic groups face additional racial discrimination, and language barriers that may impact on their living environment and economic resources thus impeding their use of health and welfare services. We have argued that minority ethnic women are particularly at risk of material and financial hardship in old age, due to their lower levels of previous employment and interrupted occupational history. The marked health disadvantage of older minority ethnic women cannot be explained by cigarette smoking, since white women have the highest level of smoking but the best reported health.

To understand more about the health of older white and minority ethnic women, research needs to address how both health and health-related behaviour are shaped by their socio-economic profile during working life and in old age. Our findings suggest socio-economic disadvantage is a main explanation for the high morbidity of minority ethnic women. Nonetheless, the utility of existing socio-economic measures such as social class, to represent the social status of older women, should continue to be critically examined, in parallel with the development of more sensitive socio-economic indicators.

Acknowledgment

We are grateful to the Health Development Agency (formerly the Health Education Authority) for access to the Black and Minority Ethnic Groups and Health and Lifestyles survey data and for funding the research on which this chapter is based.

Further reading

Bedi, R., 'Betel-quid and Tobacco Chewing among the United Kingdom's Bangladeshi Community', *British Journal of Cancer* **74** (Suppl. XXIX) (1996), S73–77.

Cooper, H., Arber, S., Daly, T., Smaje, C. and Ginn, J., *Ethnicity, Health and Health Behaviour: A Study of Older Age Groups.* (London: Health Development Agency 2000)
    URL: www.hda online.org.uk/downloads/pdfs/ethnicity_studyolder.pdf

Erens, B., Primatesta, P. and Prior, G., *Health Survey for England: The Health of Minority Ethnic Groups 1999* (London: The Stationery Office, 2000).

Ginn, J. and Arber, S., 'Ethnic Inequality in Later Life: Variation in Financial Circumstances by Gender and Ethnic Group', *Education and Ageing,* **15,** 1 (2000), 65–83.

14
Discursive Challenges: Reproductive Rights and Women's Well-Being in Developing Countries

Catherine Locke

The management of fertility, sexual relationships and child-bearing is central to women's well-being everywhere, but this link is made even more important in developing countries, where poverty and inadequate health services lead to high rates of maternal mortality and morbidity and the spread of sexually transmitted diseases, particularly HIV/AIDs. Recent contributions to the understanding of reproductive behaviour have considerably enriched debates about its relation to wider processes of social change (such as Bledsoe, 1994; Greenhalgh, 1995; McNicoll, 1994), to the experience of well-being (such as Harcourt, 1997; Petchesky and Judd, 1998), and the politics of social policy about reproduction (such as Finkle and McIntosh, 1994; Fraser, 1989; Sen et al., 1994). These often interdisciplinary interpretations, including insights from anthropology, sociology and politics, offer highly differentiated and contextualized perspectives concerned with the meaning of subjective experiences of reproduction as well as societal well-being. They are variously feminist in their politics or strongly gendered in their analyses, and seek to make linkages between local, national and global dynamics, through historically informed and institutionally situated understandings. The greater prominence of these interpretations has coincided with very real steps towards international agreement on a universal standard for reproductive well-being.

The 'Programme of Action' from the International Conference on Population and Development at Cairo in 1994 marked a dramatic victory for women's health advocates. Its affirmation that reproductive rights were human rights appeared to close the door on the population control perspectives which had dominated four decades of international discussion about social policy for reproduction, adversely affecting the ethos of family planning policies in the developing world. None the less, optimism about a new consensus must take account of multiple interpretations of reproductive rights, which create constraints as well as opportunities for reproductive rights advocates trying to improve women's well-being.

The Cairo conference established a critical link between reproductive health and reproductive rights. The language of its programme of action grounded that link in an understanding of gender and wider processes of social change. The proper objective of population and development efforts was now clearly defined as improving reproductive health in its broadest sense – 'a state of complete mental, physical and social well-being' (UN, 1994: p. 72). Although a wide range of reproductive rights could be linked to the original 1948 declaration of International Human Rights, Cairo was significant as the first time that they were coherently elaborated in the United Nations system. This endorsement emerged from the negotiations within and around the official conference between an unprecedented range of stakeholders. These included the UN agencies, national governments, family policymakers, health professionals, non-governmental organizations concerned with women's health, women's rights, population and environment and religious organizations, including the Roman Catholic Holy See and other Christian and Islamic groups.

United Nations' conferences following Cairo have reaffirmed the importance of reproductive health and of rights-based approaches to social policy (Petchesky, 2000: p. 16), and population planning. The international development targets for 2015 include cutting maternal mortality by 75 per cent and making reproductive health care universally accessible (Ferguson, 1999: pp. 35–45). A rhetorical shift towards reproductive health is widely evident in donor programming, in the activities of NGOs and in national programmes, including statements about reproductive rights.

These twin trends – the development of interdisciplinary approaches and a universal standard for reproductive health – have, in some senses, been mutually supportive but, in other senses, have raised unresolved areas of tension. This chapter examines understandings of reproductive rights in relation to women's health and well-being, asks how women's reproductive rights are interpreted in diverse circumstances and considers what they mean in the context of today's predominantly neoliberal social policy agendas. Its analysis draws on academic interdisciplinary understandings about reproductive behaviours and reproductive policies. It is argued that struggles over the meaning and content of reproductive rights can make a difference to the way in which social policy, and its implementation by health services, respond to women's interests in developing countries.

Reproductive rights and women's well-being

The reproductive rights discourse takes for granted the central relationships between reproductive rights, reproductive health and women's (reproductive) well-being. It assumes that they are mutually reinforcing and that women's well-being can be read from their 'reproductive' well-being. This discourse has focused on reproductive outcomes, such as rates for maternal survival and contraceptive use. In contrast, other strongly contextualized understandings of reproductive behaviours suggest that women's lives are more complex and that their reproductive strategies are deeply embedded in wider social processes, in ways that may well create meanings for specific outcomes which are unexpected or ambiguous (Petchesky and Judd, 1998: p. 9). Interdisciplinary approaches agree that individuals do not hold distinct reproductive goals. Rather, their reproductive behaviour and experiences are part of the 'relatively seamless whole' (Ortner, cited in Greenhalgh, 1995: p. 13).

Sex and reproduction are key strategies for forging social relationships, and sexual or reproductive 'failure' and reproductive morbidity can be overtly connected to processes of social exclusion. Women (and men) may explicitly and implicitly trade off aspects of sexual and reproductive autonomy and well-being to create room for manoeuvre in other dimensions of their lives (Petchesky and Judd, 1998: pp. 17, 19). Family and non-kin networks are sources of knowledge, skills and support for women that confer and contest the bounds of accepted sexual and reproductive behaviour (Harcourt, 1997). Institutional (McNicoll, 1994) and anthropological (Greenhalgh, 1995) approaches have explicated how reproductive health outcomes are iteratively shaped, experienced and given meaning. Social norms and practices, social policy and cultures of service provision in the management of fertility and sexuality both shape, and are shaped by, individual women's actions over time.

These insights demonstrate the value of unpacking the relationships between reproductive rights, reproductive health and women's well-being. Sen's notion of well-being, as located within the three spheres of capabilities, functionings and entitlements (Sen, 1990), usefully draws attention to the extent to which people are able to choose and achieve a range of reproductive aspirations in relation to their biological endowments. His framework aimed to shift understandings about well-being beyond the sphere of formal welfare entitlements to reproductive health services and to accommodate gender relations within and beyond the household, through the notion of 'co-operative conflicts' and 'extended entitlements'. Sen's ideas draw attention to the problems women may experience in identifying and pursuing their own well-being within the household: women's negotiation of power at home is weakened by their relative disadvantage if the household were to disintegrate and by prevailing perceptions of entitlements that put others' interests above their own.

Petchesky and Judd (1998: p. 13) develop the related concept of a 'sense of entitlement' to refer to 'moral claims, especially on partners, kin and caregivers'. Importantly, 'sense of entitlement' cannot be equated with normative morality but is grounded in the ways women act to secure what they perceive to be their own and their children's needs (1998: p. 14). Consequently, entitlement is dynamic and problematic, often displaying wide disjunctures between women's private actions and their public justifications with respect to reproduction. As a result, women's strategies to pursue the things they feel they and their children need may be manipulative and carefully concealed.

A social science perspective reveals how ideas about rights have developed over time and that particular interpretations of rights emerge from and lend themselves to specific ideologies. While upholding the view that the expansion of reproductive rights is a 'good thing', I none the less want to uncover some of the complexities of these social constructions to consider what rights-based approaches to social policy about reproduction might mean for women's well-being.

Constructing women's reproductive rights

Success in legitimizing reproductive rights stems partly from women's health activists having drawn on the women's rights agenda to 'emphasize the right to respect for bodily integrity and the concept of informed choice' (Whitty, 1996: p. 226). Whereas previous women's rights were derivative from rights extended to men, on the grounds of their being 'abstract individuals', reproductive rights focus on 'bodied individuals' and 'uniquely apply to women' (Ramirez and McEneaney, 1997: pp. 7, 10). However, the 'bodied' nature of the mainstream approach to reproductive rights is clearly embedded in notions of motherhood, heterosexuality and, to a lesser extent, links between marriage and family (Whitty, 1996: p. 227). This is demonstrated by the continuing controversy over reproductive rights for adolescents (Ramirez and McEneaney, 1997: p. 19).

The language of the programme of action recognizes the special importance of reproduction to women's lives on the grounds both of their biological endowments and their socially constructed roles. However, the woman-centred interpretation of reproductive rights also constructs men in particular ways: as uninformed, irresponsible, blocking women's contraceptive use, promiscuous and as under-investing in their children (Greene, 2000). This limited view of gender roles can reinforce gender stereotypes (Greene, 2000) and may ultimately restrict the capacity of this agenda to address women's interests.

The current concept of reproductive rights transcends the 'right to reproduce' to encompass healthful sexual and reproductive relationships and is, for the first time, strongly rooted in the context of gender equality. However, the 'bodied' interpretation of reproductive rights tends to distract attention from the broader social and material context of livelihoods. Freedman and Isaacs (1993) remind us that reproductive choice becomes meaningful only when the full constellation of rights is achieved and frame this challenge as ensuring that 'the notion of reproductive autonomy' (1993: 28) is pervasive. A narrow approach to empowerment can neglect the gendered link between material livelihoods and reproductive and sexual strategies, even though ample evidence has shown that women use their sexual and reproductive capabilities as resources in their everyday struggles, and has directly linked child sex-trafficking and commercial sex-working with poverty.

The relatively longstanding emphasis on reproductive autonomy presupposes that women make rational, or at least explicit and stable, choices about reproductive matters. While reflecting new understandings of reproductive agency, this emphasis does not engage with the ambiguity of reproductive 'choices' and their emotive and changing nature. It is now well accepted that focusing only on reproductive outcomes, such as 'births averted' or 'couple years of contraceptive protection', prejudges the meaning of reproductive experiences for women's well-being. Jain and Bruce (1994) attempt to deepen the measurement of reproductive well-being by factoring in reproductive choice, but evaluating outcomes only in terms of women's *a priori* subjective preferences incompletely describes both reproductive experiences and well-being. Discussions of reproductive agency need to engage closely with the complex relational content of 'decision-making' and the processes whereby social and cultural institutions shape 'choice', giving it meaning over time. This means that we need to take seriously women's own narratives of their experiences as they unfold, and to balance these accounts with more objective assessments of their well-being.

Interdisciplinary understandings of reproductive behaviour, therefore, raise questions about the links between reproductive rights, health and well-being as framed within the rights discourse. They draw attention to the importance of making distinctions between these concepts, stressing the relational quality of reproduction, its embeddedness in material livelihoods, and the complexity of untangling the meaning of women's reproductive experiences.

Interpreting reproductive rights in diverse circumstances

Reproductive rights are implicated in the tension between universal standards and the economic, political, social and cultural diversity that has characterized debates about international human rights since they were first declared in 1948. Formally, the framework for international human rights allows space for the local interpretation of how these rights may be best addressed. Such a framework complements the approach of human needs theorists who construct universal well-being in terms of locally specified functionings that make up a 'a good life' (Jackson, 1997: 146). The challenge of recognizing the importance of subjective well-being, without regarding it as determining, is particularly important for women whose perceptions and priorities are powerfully shaped by gendered power relations that can 'naturalize' ill-being and altruism. Recent human needs theory has provided a basis for defending women's *critical* autonomy to make well-being choices for themselves, where they have knowledge of alternative courses of action, thus balancing concerns about women's rights and their human needs (Doyal and Gough, 1991).

Rights discourse is rooted in Western liberal individualism and rights standards are often applied in ethnocentric ways. However, recent feminist emphasis on difference and diversity has 'opened the door for a redefinition of rights that is more conducive to dialogue' (Obermeyer, 1995: 367), and social movements worldwide have utilized the language of rights to make claims to social justice (Ferguson, 1999; Gloppen and Rakner, 1993). The advocacy of Southern women's groups has influenced the meaning of reproductive rights, and their contribution in linking women's reproductive health to a comprehensive human development framework has proved particularly significant in ensuring that the interests of women in developing countries are better articulated (Correa and Reichmann, 1994; Petchesky, 2000: p. 3).

Despite women's groups from different places having different agendas to prioritize in relation to reproductive rights, the emerging maturity of the networks between women's health movements, and particularly their creation of women's coalitions to lobby the United Nations' conferences, has enabled a shared vision of fundamental rights (Petchesky, 2000: pp. 4–5).

The International Reproductive Rights Research Action Group's enquiry into the everyday ways in which women negotiate reproductive health and sexual matters explored what reproductive and sexual rights might mean to women in seven countries across the globe (Petchesky and Judd, 1998). Despite evidence that women's perceptions were influenced in complex ways by prevailing power relations, their findings clearly supported a universal ethical core that can provide a sound basis for reproductive rights. 'Most of our respondents in all seven countries showed a clear sense of entitlement to make their own decisions with regard to marriage (when and to whom), fertility (number and timing of children), contraception, avoidance of domestic violence and unwanted sex, child care and work' (1998: p. 316) and they justified this sense of reproductive entitlement in motherhood. There is overwhelming evidence of 'women's determination in all eras, countries and cultures to seek abortions, even at great risk to their lives and health, in order to gain some control over their fertility and bodies' (Petchesky, 2000: 17). This work on shared ethical values is supported by investigations of cross-cultural perceptions of rights. For example, Obermeyer (1993: 366) explores the commonalities between notions of reproductive rights in the Western tradition and the principles that define gender rights in Islam.

While strengthening the idea of an ethical core for universal rights on the basis of philosophy, theorizing, advocacy and the everyday aspirations and strategies of women, we still 'need to examine much more closely what we really mean by an individual human right to reproductive choice, freedom, or autonomy in a world as demographically complex and culturally diverse as ours' (Freedman and Isaacs, 1993: 18). Considerable progress has been made in this respect within a growing literature of women's visions and strategies for change in developing countries. However, with a few notable exceptions, relatively little attention has been given to the process of interpreting rights in diverse circumstances in international social policy, in donor policy and activity, or in national social policy and provisioning. One exception is Brazil where an institutionalized 'partnership' has evolved between the national women's health movement and the government.

Another exception is action by government agencies responsible for implementing the Cairo programme of action, which has led to substantial policy and legislative reforms and giving women's health advocates an official voice in planning and monitoring reproductive health policy and service provision (Petchesky, 2000: 40–1). Also notable is the success of the International Planned Parenthood Federation, whose Charter on Sexual and Reproductive Rights was developed using a detailed review process enabling direct input from member associations which makes plain the connections between human rights language and service delivery (Newman and Helzner, 1999: p. 459).

These discursive views of rights create space for diverse interpretations of rights but practical politics means that such negotiability can be used to undermine their radicalism. Ramirez and McEneaney's (1997) study of the liberalization of abortion laws concluded that gains in reproductive rights were reversible and poorly institutionalized. There can be no complacency over the apparent legitimation of reproductive rights. This was evident in the United Nations' five-year review of progress since the Cairo Conference, when debates about fundamental principles were reopened (Petchesky, 2000: p. 30) and in President Bush's retraction, immediately on entering office in 2001, of US overseas assistance funds for programmes supporting abortion.

The Cairo Conference, while expanding the boundaries of reproductive rights, builds in various compromises accommodating the broad range of interpretations underlying its consensus. These include careful wording around contested issues, conflating the terms 'individuals' and 'couples', justifying the language of 'responsibility' and explicitly circumventing discussion of abortion rights (UN, 1994). Its Programme of Action's right to reproduce 'freely' is assigned to 'individuals and all couples' and remains contingent on the obligation to do so 'responsibly' (UN, 1994: p. 7.3). The balance of power between individuals and couples is not fully explored, creating space for pressing reproductive and sexual obligations within marital partnerships. 'Responsibly' is not defined, thus keeping the door open for expert and elite judgements about what is in society's interest as well as in the best interests of the individual and her (potential) child (Ramirez and McEneaney, 1997: p. 19). Adolescents are ascribed reproductive health needs rather than rights. Although their full involvement in 'appropriate' services is upheld, it is contingent on 'appropriate regard for parental guidance and responsibility' (UN, 1994: pp. 7.44, 7.47). The Programme of Action falls short of establishing a right to abortion, but does instruct governments to make abortion safe where it is legal and, where it is not, to treat complications arising from illegal abortion. These compromises reveal the struggle with fundamentalist perspectives on women's authority over sexual and reproductive decisions, and their perceived implications for family relations (Petchesky, 2000: p. 16).

Ironically, the very success of Cairo has enabled discussions about reproductive rights to be largely contained within arenas concerned with reproductive health policy and programming. The Conference's mainstreaming of the language of empowerment has diluted its transformative intention and many argue, with reason, that this language has been used in an instrumentalist and opportunistic way. This 'enclaving' (Fraser, 1989) of reproductive rights talk within reproductive health forums has a depoliticizing function that can narrow the scope of reproductive rights and preclude innovative responses to women's reproductive interests in diverse circumstances. The implications of a rights-based approach are frequently seen unproblematically as implying a specific minimum constellation of services and attention to improving quality, particularly client-provider relationships and informed consent. In this interpretation, the Programme of Action becomes merely 'a guide on 'how to do family planning better' (Greene, 2000: p. 50).

In some instances, dialogue is being built between reproductive policy and programming and women's civil society institutions, even extending to legal reforms and broader gender policies. These consultative processes are, however, constrained by silences around reproductive problems that are intimate, taboo, or emotionally fraught (Harcourt, 1997) and beset by strongly gendered problems of stakeholder hierarchies of power. Breaking debates out of the arena of reproductive policy and programming is both necessary and dangerous: the emotive, controversial and private nature of reproduction and sexual relations has sometimes made the politicizing of reproductive issues a hostage to other agendas, often conservative. However, a 'dual political strategy' (Doyal and Gough, 1991) that effectively combines the neutrality of state-led social policy (which can defend universalized provision) with the politics of democratic participation (which can give voice to different interests) has the potential to link reproductive rights with social rights in a way that institutionalizes women's entitlements and allows for dynamic negotiation.

Reproductive rights and globalized social policy agendas

The rise of rights-based approaches to social policy, including reproductive rights, has emerged in an era of increasing globalization.

However, universally agreed social standards have, paradoxically, been agreed in a context of widespread economic crisis. One consequence has been a discursive shift in the meaning and contents of social rights. Reform strategies, including health sector reform, have reduced the scope of entitlements by shifting to minimal levels of support, by targeting beneficiaries, and by discouraging uptake: even where they remain universal, changing social policy assumptions have ensured rights are seen more as needs (Cox, 1998: pp. 6–8). Reproductive rights have, indeed, been seen within global social policy largely in terms of reproductive health needs, and it has become clear that revisionist neo-liberal perspectives and associated health sector reform strategies were strongly reflected and largely uncontested in the Cairo Programme of Action (Petchesky, 2000). The market-orientation of its implementation chapters reflects neo-liberal reforms with its references to 'cost-effectiveness', 'cost-recovery', user fees, social marketing and the promotion of the private sector (Petchesky, 2000: 19).

The broader economic agenda directly threatens progress on repro-ductive rights by undermining the universalism of health systems in developing countries and shifting the burden and cost of caring back to women and their families. Indirectly, but no less significantly, adjustment and reform processes have, in many cases, undermined the livelihoods on which women's well-being is premised, in turn leading to more risky reproductive and sexual behaviour (ranging from reduced health-seeking behaviour to commercial sex-working) and such reforms have been widely seen as undermining the authority and accountability of national governments. Reform itself is not, here, in question; what is being questioned is the way it is pursued, its values, objectives and its accountability.

Comparative analysis by social policy theorists has begun to draw out differences in the institutional context of social welfare in develop-ing countries where social institutions, especially community, family and household, are especially important for women's well-being (compare Kabeer and Cook, 2000). This points directly to the impor-tance of social movements in creating progressive social change and recognizes the limited resources of developing nation states. Literature on grassroots women's movements and reproductive rights goes beyond simply documenting women's complex realities to show how women are trying to change their lives and are identifying strategies for action and advocacy. For example, Mirsky and Radlett's (2000) contributors describe the work of women's networks in campaigning for change, enforcing standards, coordinating alliances and raising awareness. The processes of globalization have enhanced the capacity of the women's health movement to build and use transnational alliances to exert pressure to change official policies. Women's health organizations are well placed to implement rights-based approaches, but doing so potentially undermines the responsibilities of governments.

Theories of global social policy which can also be used to infer other important arenas for action for reproductive rights include: the social regulation of capital; the international redistribution of resources; and the strengthening of national accountability for social rights within a global framework (Deacon et al., 1997).

The social regulation of capital needs to be firmly linked to the reproductive rights agenda. The importance of multinational research, development and production of technologies for reproductive health (Fathalla, 1994), the growing privatization of services. whether non-governmental or commercial (Deacon, 2000), the evidence that international capital infringes reproductive rights in labour practices (Pearson and Seyfang, 2001), the trend towards corporate welfarism that ties social rights to employment, and the growing internationalism of the sex trade are just some of the reasons why this is the case.

International inequalities imply a need to redistribute resources between nations if rights concepts are to be applied in places where resources are severely constrained. Concern for reproductive rights in this forum needs to go much further than lobbying for increased donor commitment to implementing basic reproductive health care in developing countries (compare Conley and de Silva, 1998). Relying on such an approach neglects to situate reproductive rights within the context of international debt, fails to question donor motivations with respect to reproductive health and overlooks the erosion of local governance which increasing disbursements may exacerbate.

The core institutions that are responsible for delineating and monitoring rights are disproportionately influenced by Western powers; there are growing calls for their political reform and particularly for an end to the privileged role of the Roman Catholic Holy See in the UN. The international framework for accountability is being developed through the treaty monitoring committee for the Convention for the Elimination of Discrimination Against Women but is so far not linked to systems of national accountability under which individual grievances could be raised. Multidimensional approaches to monitoring, and pressuring for targets, are likely to be more successful in opening up basic standards of provision in developing country situations than simply extending the international legal framework. Such approaches

might include: submitting 'shadow' country reports to the treaty monitoring committees; lobbying governments, donors, professional associations and international institutions; using global alliances as well as
building national advocacy networks and social movements.

The World Summit for Social Development at Copenhagen in 1995
promoted a 'social integrationist' agenda. Together with the vision of
some development agencies, including the UK's Department for
International Development, this can be seen as a progressive attempt
to revitalize social rights in an attempt to bring together human
rights concerns with the concerns of the new poverty agenda (see
Hausermann, 1998; UN, 1995). These 'integrationist' perspectives are
attempting to promote a rights-based approach that focuses on social
justice and which defends basic primary education and health, including reproductive health, for all, free at the point of delivery. These
views are in tension with the currently dominant revisionist neoliber-
alism that emphasizes the privatization and marketization of education
and health and which targets the poorest in society for special assistance. However, the attempt by the World Bank and latterly the UN, to
distil 'universally agreed principles of social policy' is significant
because it defends universalized access to primary social services and
represents an opportunity to link the goals of the Copenhagen summit
to the negotiation of structural adjustment and sector reform programmes with international financial institutions (Norton, 2000).
Mainstream interpretations of reproductive rights have yet to engage
with the language of social exclusion and social integration that
characterizes these attempts to enhance the social justice of global
economic policy-making.

Shaping a reproductive rights discourse for social policy

There is scope for the emergence of a reproductive rights agenda not
only to signal the death knell of population control ethics in reproductive health services but also to ensure that social policy about reproduction addresses women's well-being. The normalization of
reproductive rights discourse has constructed women's reproductive
needs in ways that are often narrow, simplistic and insensitive to
different economic, political, social and cultural contexts. However,
the legitimation of concepts of reproductive rights has created a clear
basis for women at all levels to struggle over the meaning and contents
of a reproductive rights agenda. Advocacy, from the grassroots to
women's global networks, and feminist academic endeavour and policy
analysis, plays an ongoing role in this discursive arena and can shape

the way in which rights-based approaches address women's interests. The analysis above suggests opportunities for reinvigorating the universal ethical basis of reproductive rights whilst deepening understanding of the embedded and diverse nature of women's interests.

First, there is a need to extend situation-specific audits of reproductive rights and health to address adequately the multiple dimensions of reproductive entitlements, reproductive health outcomes and their meaning for different women's well-being. Second, we need to problematize both the interpretation of women's reproductive rights and their translation into needs, policies and services in different contexts. In this volume, Hewson, Savage, Nightingale, and Mugford and McFarlane make contributions to both these objectives in their respective chapters on Caesareans, choice in childbirth, cervical screening for women with learning disabilities, and maternity services. Third, it is necessary to understand how different women's reproductive and sexual strategies, including their health-seeking behaviour, is influenced by wider social, cultural and economic conditions. Also in this volume, Cooper and Arber write about the differences that older women experience in acting for their own health. Fourth, we need to extend the debate about reproductive rights beyond reproductive service provision and to promote dialogue about social policy globally, nationally and locally. Understandings that go beyond both expert medical opinion and women's subjective preferences, to include the insights from interdisciplinary research, can offer accounts that are sensitive to the realities of women's lives in different contexts. Together with women's advocacy, such understandings can help generate a more radical interpretation of rights-based approaches to reproduction.

Further reading

Petchesky, R.P. and K. Judd (eds), *Negotiating Reproductive Rights: Women's Perspective Across Countries and Cultures* (London: Zed, 1998).

Presser, H.B. and G. Sen (eds), *Women's Empowerment and Demographic Processes: Moving Beyond Cairo* (Oxford: Oxford University Press, 2000).

Sen, G. and C.R. Snow (eds), *Power and Decision: The Social Control of Reproduction* (Boston: Harvard University Press, 1994).

SID (The Society for International Development), *Development*, 42 (1) (1999). (This issue is edited by Wendy Harcourt and focuses on reproductive health and rights.)

References

Abbott, P., *An Introduction to Sociology: Feminist Perspectives* (London: Routledge, 1990).

Adams, P., 'Toward a Family Support Approach with Drug-using Parents: The Importance of Social Worker Attitudes and Knowledge', *Social Work Review*, 8 (1999) 15–28.

Ahmad, W.I.U. and Walker, R., 'Asian Older People: Housing, Health and Access to Services', *Ageing and Society*, 17 (1997) 141–65.

Ahmad, W.I.U., 'Making Black People Sick: "Race", Ideology and Health Research', in W.I.U. Ahmad (ed.), *'Race' and Health in Contemporary Britain* (Buckingham: Open University Press, 1993).

Ahmad, W.I.U., 'The Trouble with Culture' in D. Kelleher and S. Hillier (eds), *Researching Cultural Differences in Health* (London: Routledge, 1996).

Ainscough, C. and Toon, K., *Breaking Free* (London: Sheldon Press, 2000).

ALBSU (Adult Literacy and Basic Skills Unit) *Literacy, Numeracy and Adults – Evidence from the Child Development Study* (London: ALBSU, 1987).

Alexander, P.C., 'Application of Attachment Theory to the Study of Sexual Abuse', *Journal of Consulting and Clinical Psychology*, 60 (1992) 185–95.

Allen, C., 'Helping with Deliberate Self-Harm: Some Practical Guidelines', *Journal of Mental Health*, 4 (1995) 243–50.

Al-Mufti, R., McCarthy, A. and Fisk, N.M., 'Obstetricians' Personal Choice and Mode of Delivery', *Lancet*, 347 (1996) 544.

American Psychiatric Association, *Statistical Diagnosis of Mental Disorders*, 3rd revised edn (Washington: APA, 1987).

American Psychiatric Association, *Diagnostic and Statistical Manual of Mental Disorders*, 4th edn (Washington: APA, 1994).

Amir, G., 'Au menu de Vital: Un concentre d'idéologie de rapport aux sport', in *Sport et changement social. Actes des premières journées d'études* (Bordeaux: Maison des sciences de l'homme d'Aquitaine, 1987).

Anthias, A. and Yuval-Davis, N., 'Connecting Race and Gender', in F. Anthias and N. Yuval-Davis (eds), *Racialized Boundaries* (London: Routledge, 1992).

Apple, M., *You and Your Doctor: The Essential Guide to Examinations, Tests and Investigations* (Oxford: Oxford University Press, 1997).

Arber, S. and Cooper, H., 'Gender and Inequalities in Health across the Lifecourse', in E. Annandale and K. Hunt (eds), *Gender Inequalities in Health* (Buckingham: Open University Press, 1999).

Audit Commission, *Seen but not Heard* (London: HMSO, 1994).

Audit Commission, *First Class Delivery: Improving Maternity Services in England and Wales* (London: Audit Commission, 1997).

Audit Commission, *Children in Mind* (London: HMSO, 1999).

Baer, M., Marlatt, G.A. and McMahon, M. (eds), *Addictive Behaviours across the Lifespan: Prevention, Treatment and Policy Issues* (California: Sage, 1981).

Bagley, C. and Ramsey, R., 'Sexual Abuse in Childhood: Psychological Outcomes and Implications for Social Work Practice', *Journal of Social Work and Human Sexuality*, 5 (1986) 33–47.

Bainham, A., *Children – The Modern Law* (Bristol: Family Law, 1998).

Baldessarini, R.J., *Chemotherapy in Psychiatry: Principles and Practice* (Cambridge, MA: Harvard University Press, 1985).

Barnett, R. and Marshall, N., 'The Relationship between Women's Work and Family Roles and their Subjective Well-being and Psychological Distress', in M. Frankenhaeuser, U. Lundberg and M. Chesney (eds), *Women, Work and Health: Stress and Opportunities* (New York: Plenum Press, 1991).

Bartley, M., Popay, J. and Plewis, J., 'Domestic Conditions, Paid Employment and Women's Experiences of Ill Health', *Sociology of Health and Illness*, 14 (3) (1992) 313–41.

Battison, G., Todd, C. and Morgan, K., 'Models of Helping and Coping among Parasuicides and Hospital Staff' (Ipswich Hospitals: unpublished research, 1993).

Beard, G.M., *American Nervousness: Its Causes and Consequences, a Supplement to Nervous Exhaustion (Neurasthenia)* (New York: Arno Press, 1972 [1881]).

Beardow, R., Oerton, J. and Victor, C., 'Evaluation of the Cervical Cytology Screening Programme in an Inner City Health District', *British Medical Journal*, 299 (1989) 98–100.

Beck, A.T., *Depression: Clinical, Experimental and Theoretical Aspects* (New York: Harper and Row, 1967).

Beck, A.T., *Cognitive Therapy and Emotional Disorders* (New York: International Universities Press, 1976).

Beck, A.T., 'Cognitive Therapy: A 30-year Retrospective'. *American Psychologist*, 46 (4) (1991) 368–75.

Beck, A.T., Epstein, N., Brown, G. and Steer, A., 'An Inventory for Measuring Clinical Anxiety: Psychometric Properties', *Journal of Consulting and Clinical Psychology*, 56 (6) (1988) 893–7.

Beck, A.T., Ward, C.H., Mendelson, M., Mock, J.E. and Erbaugh, J.K., 'An Inventory for Measuring Depression', *Archives of General Psychiatry*, 4 (1961) 561–71.

Beck, J.S., *Cognitive Therapy: Basics and Beyond* (New York: Guilford Press, 1995).

Bedi, R., 'Betel-quid and Tobacco Chewing among the United Kingdom's Bangladeshi Community', *British Journal of Cancer*, 74 (Supplement XXIX) (1996) S73–7.

Beitchman, J.H., Zucker, K.J., Hood, J.E., DaCosta, G.A. and Cassavia, E., 'A Review of the Long-term Effects of Child Sexual Abuse', *Child Abuse and Neglect*, 16 (1992) 101–18.

Belle, D., 'Poverty and Women's Mental Health', *American Psychologist*, 45 (1990) 385–89.

Bendelow, G. and Williams, S.J., *Emotions in Social Life: Critical Themes and Social Issues* (London: Routledge, 1998).

Berryman, J., 'Exercise and the Medical Tradition from Hippocrates through Antebellum America', in J. Berryman and R. Park (eds), *Sport and Exercise Science: Essays in the History of Sport Medicine* (Urbana: University of Illinois Press, 1992).

Bird, C.E. and Rieker, P.P., 'Gender Matters: An Integrated Model for Understanding Men's and Women's Health', *Social Science and Medicine*, 48 (1999) 745–55.

Blake, W., *Complete Writings of William Blake* (Oxford, New York: Oxford University Press, 1966).

Blakemore, K. and Boneham, M., *Age, Race and Ethnicity: A Comparative Approach* (Buckingham: Open University Press, 1994).

Blaxter, M. *Health and Lifestyles* (London: Tavistock/Routledge, 1990).

Bledsoe, C., '"Children are like young bamboo trees": Potentiality and Reproduction in Sub-Saharan Africa', in K. Lindahl-Kiessling and H. Landberg (eds), *Population, Economic Development, and the Environment* (Oxford: Oxford University Press, 1994).

Bloor, M., 'A User's Guide to Contrasting Theories of HIV-related Risk Behaviour', in J. Gabe (ed.), *Medicine, Health and Risk* (Oxford: Blackwell, 1995).

Bordo, S., *Unbearable Weight. Feminism, Western Culture and the Body* (Berkeley: University of California Press, 1993).

Boseley, S., 'To Screen or not to Screen', *The Guardian* (16 March 1999), 14.

Boserup, E., *Women's Role in Economic Development* (London: George Allen and Unwin, 1970).

Boswell, G.R., *Young and Dangerous: The Backgrounds and Careers of Section 53 Offenders* (Aldershot: Avebury, 1996).

Botting, B.J., Macfarlane, A.J. and Price, F.V., *Three, Four and More: A National Survey of Triplet and Higher Order Births* (London: HMSO, 1990).

Bourdieu, P., 'Sport and Social Class', *Social Science Information*, 17 (6) (1978) 819–40.

Bowlby, J., *Attachment and Loss, vol. 1* (Harmondsworth: Penguin, 1971).

Bowlby, J., *Separation: Anxiety and Anger – Attachment and Loss, vol. 2* (Harmondsworth: Penguin, 1975).

Bowlby, J., *Loss, Sadness and Depression – Attachment and Loss, vol. 3* (Harmondsworth: Penguin, 1980).

Bowlby, J., *The Making and Breaking of Affectional Bonds* (Oxford: Penguin, 1991).

Breggin, P., *Toxic Psychiatry – Drugs and Electroconvulsive Therapy: The Truth and the Better Alternative* (London: HarperCollins, 1993).

Brems, S. and Griffiths, M., 'Health Women's Way: Learning to Listen', in M. Koblinsky, J. Timyan and J. Gay, *The Health of Women: A Global Perspective* (Boulder, CO: Westview Press, 1993).

Brennan, P.A., Hammen, C., Andersen, M.J., Bor, W., Najman, J.M. and Williams, G.M., 'Chronicity, Severity and Timing of Maternal Depressive Symptoms: Relationships with Child Outcomes at age 5', *Developmental Psychology*, 36 (6) (2000) 759–66.

Brennan, T., *The Interpretation of the Flesh: Freud and Femininity* (London: Routledge, 1992).

Brenner, H., *Mental Health and the Economy* (Cambridge, MA: Harvard University Press, 1978).

Briere, J.N., *Child Abuse Trauma. Theory and Treatment of the Lasting Effects* (London: Sage, 1992).

Brockington, I.F. and Kumar, R. (eds), *Motherhood and Mental Illness* (London: Academic Press, 1982).

Brown, G. and Harris, T., *Social Origins of Depression* (London: Tavistock, 1978).

Brown, H., 'Abuse of Adults with Learning Difficulties', *Nursing Standard*, 6 (26) (1992) 18–19.

Buckley, K., 'Managing Violence: Managing Masculinity', in H. Kemshall and J. Pritchard (eds), *Good Practice in Working with Violence* (London; Philadelphia: Jessica Kingsley, 1999).

Buckley, R. and Bigelow, D.A., 'The Multi-service Network: Reaching the Unserved Multi-problem Individual', *Community Mental Health Journal,* 28 (1) (1992) 43–50.

Bureau of International Labor Affairs, *Forced Labor: The Prostitution of Children* (Washington: US Department of Labor, 1996).

Bureau of International Labor Affairs, *By the Sweat and Toil of Children* (Washington: US Department of Labor, 1998).

Burstow, B., *Radical Feminist Therapy: Working in the Context of Violence* (London: Sage, 1992).

Burt, M.R. and Katz, B.L., 'Dimensions of Recovery from Rape: Focus on Growth Outcomes', *Journal of Interpersonal Violence,* 2 (1987) 55–82.

Busfield, J., 'The Female Malady? Men, Women and Madness in Nineteenth-century Britain', *Sociology,* 28 (1994) 259–77.

Busfield, J., *Men, Women and Madness: Understanding Gender and Mental Disorder* (London: Macmillan, 1996).

Busfield, J., 'The Archaeology of Psychiatric Disorder: Gender and Disorders of Thought, Emotion and Behaviour', in G. Bendelow, M. Carpenter, C. Vautier and S. Williams (eds), *Gender, Health and Healing: the Public/Private Divide* (London: Routledge, 2002).

Butler, G., *Manage Your Mind* (Oxford: Oxford University Press, 1995).

Butterworth, T., *Working in Partnership* (London: HMSO, 1994)

Cadden, J., *Meanings of Sex Difference in the Middle Ages* (Cambridge: Cambridge University Press, 1993).

Cahill, C., Llewelyn, S.P. and Pearson, C., 'Long-term Effects of Sexual Abuse which Occurred in Childhood: A Review', *British Journal of Clinical Psychology,* 30 (1991) 117–30.

Callender, C., Millward, N., Lissenburgh, S. and Forth, J., *Maternity Rights and Benefits in Britain 1996,* DSS research report no. 67 (London: The Stationery Office, 1997).

Calvino, I., *Our Ancestors* (London: Picador 1980).

Campbell, J., Rose, L., Kub, J., and Nedd, D., 'Voices of Strength and Resistance; A Contextual and Longitudinal Analysis of Women's Responses to Battering', *Journal of Interpersonal Violence,* 13 (6) (1998) 743–62.

Campbell, J.C. and Socken, K.L., 'Women's Responses to Battering over Time: An Analysis of Change', *Journal of Interpersonal Violence,* 14 (1) (1999) 21–40.

Campbell, J.C., *Assessing Dangerousness: Violence by Sexual Offenders, Batterers and Child Abusers* (Newbury Park, CA: Sage, 1995).

Campbell, R. and Macfarlane, A., *Where to be Born? The Debate and the Evidence* (Oxford: NPEU, 1st edn 1987; 2nd edn 1994).

Campbell, R., Davies, I.M., Macfarlane, A. and Beral, V., 'Home Births in England and Wales 1979', *British Medical Journal,* 289 (1983) 721–4.

Campbell, S.B., Cohn, J.F. and Meyers, T.A., 'Depression in First-time Mothers: Mother–Infant Interaction and Depression Chronicity', *Developmental Psychology,* 31 (1995) 349–57.

Carmen, E.H. and Rieker, P., 'A Psychosocial Model of the Victim-to-Patient Process', *Psychiatric Clinics of North America,* 12(2) (1989) 431–43.

Celentano, D., Shediac, M., Crosby, C., Mamon, J., Sanders, B. and Matanoski, G., 'Adequacy of Cervical Cancer Screening Among Inner City Women: Results from a Defined Population', *Health Education Research*, 4 (4) (1989) 451–60.

Chalmers, I., Enkin, M. and Keirse, M., (eds), *Effective Care in Pregnancy and Childbirth* (Oxford: Oxford University Press, 1989).

Chamberlain, G., Wright, A. and Crowley, P., *Home Births: The Report of the 1994 Confidential Enquiry by the National Birthday Trust Fund* (Carnforth, Lancs: Parthenon, 1996).

Chervenak F. et al., 'An Ethical Justification for Emergency, Coerced Caesarean Delivery', *Obstetrics and Gynaecology*, 82 (1993) 1029.

Chesney-Lind, M., *The Female Offender: Girls, Women and Crime* (London: Page, 1997).

CIIR (Catholic Institute for International Relations), *HIV/AIDS in Southern Africa: The Threat to Development* (London: Russell Press, 1999).

Clark D.M. and Fairburn, C.G., *Science and Practice of Cognitive Behaviour Therapy* (Oxford: Oxford University Press, 1997).

Clark, D.M., 'A Cognitive Approach to Panic', *Behaviour Research and Therapy*, 24 (1986) 461–70.

Clark, D.M., 'A Cognitive Model of Panic Attacks', in S. Rachman and J.D. Maser (eds), *Panic: Psychological Perspectives* (Hillsdale, NJ: Lawrence Erlbaum, 1988)

Clark, S.C. and Taffel, S.M., 'Rates of Caesarean and VBAC delivery, United States 1994', *Birth*, 23 (1996) 166–8.

Clarke, L. and Whittaker, M., 'Self-mutilation: Culture, Contexts and Nursing Responses', *Journal of Advanced Nursing*, 7 (1998) 129–37.

Cochrane Collaboration (The) (The Cochrane Library, Oxford: Update Software, 2000).

Cohen, P., 'Balancing Act', *Social Work Today*, 22 (1990) 18–19.

Cole, P.M. and Putman, F.W., 'Effects of Incest on Self and Social Functioning: A Developmental Psychopathology Perspective', *Journal of Consulting and Clinical Psychology*, 60 (1992) 174–84.

Coleman, L. and Dickinson, C., 'The Risks of Healing: The Hazards of the Nursing Profession', in W. Chavkin (ed.), *Double Exposure: Women's Health Hazards on the Job and at Home* (New York: Monthly Review Press, 1984).

Committee on Child Health Services Report, *Fit for the Future* [Chair, S.D.M. Court], Cmnd 6684, Vol. I (London: HMSO, 1976).

Conley S.R. and de Silva, S., *Paying Their Fair Share? Donor Countries and International Population Assistance* (Washington DC: PAI, 1998).

Cook D.J. and Allan, C.A., 'Stressful Life-events and Alcohol Abuse in Women: A General Population Study', *British Journal of Addiction*, 79 (1984) 425–30.

Cook, R., *Women's Health and Human Rights: The Promotion and Protection of Women's Health through International Human Rights Law* (Geneva: World Health Organisation, 1994).

Cooper, H., Arber S. and Ginn J., *Health-related Behaviour and Attitudes of Older People* (London: Health Education Authority, 1999).

Cooper, H., Arber, S., Daly, T., Smaje C. and Ginn, J., *Ethnicity, Health and Health Behaviour: A Study of Older Age Groups* (London: Health Development Agency, 2000). URL: www.hda-online.org.uk/downloads/pdfs/ethnicity_studyolder.pdf.

Corbin, W.R., Bernat, J.A., Calbourn, K.S., McNair L.D. and Seals, R., 'The Role of Alcohol Expectancies and Alcohol Consumption among Sexually Victimised and Nonvictimised College Women', *Journal of Interpersonal Violence*, 16 (4) (2001) 297–311.

Correa, S.S. and Reichmann, R.L., *Population and Reproductive Rights: Feminist Perspectives from the South* (London: Zed, 1994).

Courtois, C., 'The Incest Experience and its Aftermath', *Victimology: An International Journal*, 4 (1979) 337–47.

Cox, A.D., C. Puckering, C., Pound, A. and Mills, M., 'The Impact of Maternal Depression in Young Children', *Child Psychology and Psychiatry*, 28 (6) (1987) 917–28.

Cox, R.H., 'The Consequences of Welfare Reform: How Conceptions of Social Rights are Changing', *Journal of Social Policy*, 27 (1) (1998) 1–16.

Crawford, R. 'A Cultural Account of Health – Self-control, Release and Social Body', in J. McKinlay (ed.), *Issues in the Political Economy of Health Care* (New York: Methuen, 1985).

Crittenden, P.M., 'Quality of Attachment in the Pre-School Years', *Development and Psychopathology*, 4 (1992) 209–41.

Cummings, E.M. and P.T. Davies, P.T., 'Maternal Depression and Child Development', *Journal of Child Psychology and Psychiatry*, 35 (1) (1994) 73–112.

Dace, E., Faulkner, A., Frost, M., Parker, K., Pembroke, L. and Smith, A., *The Hurt Yourself Less Workbook* (London: National Self Harm Network, 1998).

Dally, A., *Women under the Knife: A History of Surgery* (London: Hutchinson, 1991).

Daniels, C.R., *At Women's Expense: State Power and the Politics of Fetal Rights* (Cambridge, Mass: Harvard University Press, 1993).

DAWN, *Survey of Facilities for Women Using Drugs including Alcohol* (London: DAWN, 1994).

Deacon, B., 'Globalisation: A Threat to Equitable Social Provision?', *IDS Bulletin*, 31 (4) (2000) 32–41.

Deacon, B., Hulse, M. and Stubbs, P., *Global Social Policy: International Organisations and the Future of Welfare* (London: Sage, 1997).

DeBruin, D., 'Justice and the Inclusion of Women in Clinical Studies: A Conceptual Framework', in A. Mastroianni, R. Faden and D. Federman (eds), *Women and Health Research: Ethical and Legal Issues of Including Women in Clinical Studies* (Washington DC: National Academy Press, 1994).

Declercq, E., 'Changing Childbirth in the United Kingdom: Lessons for U.S. Health Policy', *Journal of Health Politics, Policy and Law*, 23 (5) (1998) 833–59.

Declercq, E. and Viisainen, K., 'The Politics of Numbers: The Promise and Frustration of Cross-national Analysis', in R. DeVries, C. Benoit, E. van Teijlingen, S. Wrede (eds), *Birth by Design: Maternity Care and Midwifery in North America and Europe* (New York: Routledge, 2001).

Department of Health, *The Children Act 1989; Guidance and Regulations Vol. 2* (London: HMSO, 1989).

Department of Health, *The Care of Children: Principles and Practice in Regulations and Guidance* (London: HMSO, 1991).

Department of Health, Letter re; NHS Cervical Cancer Screening Programme; Personal collection (1992).

Department of Health, *The Patient's Charter* (London: HMSO, 1992).

Department of Health, *Health and Personal Social Services Statistics for England*, 1992 edition (London: HMSO, 1992).

Department of Health, *Changing Childbirth Part I. Report of the Expert Maternity Group* [Cumberledge Report] (London: HMSO, 1993).

Department of Health, *Children in Need* (London: HMSO, 1996).

Department of Health, *Messages from Research: Meeting the Needs of the Children of Depressed Mothers* (London, HMSO, 1996).

Department of Health, *Working Together* (London: HMSO, 1999).

Department of Health (DH), Welsh Office, Scottish Office Home and Health Department, Department of Health and Social Services, Northern Ireland, *Confidential Enquiries into Maternal Deaths in the United Kingdom 1994–96* (London: HMSO, 1998).

Department of Health and Human Services, *Healthy People 2000* (Washington, DC: DHSS Pub. No.[PHS] 91: 50212, 1991).

Desjarlais, R., Eisenberg, L., Good, B. and Kleinman, A., *World Mental Health: Problems and Priorities in Low-Income Countries* (Oxford: Oxford University Press, 1995).

DFID (Department for International Development), *Justice and Poverty Reduction* (London; Glasgow: DFID, 2000).

DHSS (Department of Health and Social Security) *Health Service Development: Cervical Cytology Recall Scheme*, HN (81) 14 Health Notice (April, 1981a).

DHSS (Department of Health and Social Security) *Health Service Development: Cervical Cytology Recall Scheme*, HC (81) Health Circular (14 December 1981b).

DHSS (Department of Health and Social Security) *Health Service Management: Cervical Screening*, HC (88) 1 HC (FP) (88) 2 Health Circular (January 1988).

DHSS (Department of Health and Social Security), *Confidential Enquiry into Maternal Deaths in England and Wales 1982–4* (London: HMSO, 1989).

Dinnerstein M. and Weitz, R., 'Jane Fonda, Barbara Bush and Other Aging Bodies: Femininity and the Limits of Resistance', in R. Weitz (ed.), *The Politics of Women's Bodies* (Oxford: Oxford University Press, 1998).

Djuretic, T., Laing-Morton, T., Guy, M., 'Cervical Screening for Women with Learning Disability: Concerted Effort is Needed to Ensure these Women Use Preventative Services', *British Medical Journal*, 318 (1999) 537.

Donnelly, L., 'Wired for Sound', *Health Service Journal*, 110 (2000) 5961: 18.

Donnison, J., *Midwives and Medical Men* (New York: Schocken Books, 1977).

Dowd, J. and Bengston, V., 'Ageing in Minority Populations: An Examination of the Double Jeopardy Hypothesis', *Journal of Gerontology*, 33 (3) (1978) 427–36.

Downey G. and Coyne, J.C., 'Children of Depressed Parents: An Integrative Review', *Psychological Bulletin*, 108 (1990) 50–76.

Doy, R., 'Women who Self-Harm and the Women who Care for Them' (unpublished MA thesis, Cambridge: Anglia Polytechnic University, 1995).

Doyal, L., 'Women and the National Health Service: The Carers and the Careless', in E. Lewin and V. Olesen (eds), *Women, Health and Healing: Toward a New Perspective* (London: Tavistock, 1985).

Doyal, L. and Gough, I., *A Theory of Human Need* (Basingstoke: Macmillan Education, 1991).

Doyal, L., *What Makes Women Sick* (Basingstoke: Macmillan, 1995).

Doyal, L., 'Gender Equity in Health: Debates and Dilemmas', *Social Science and Medicine*, 51 (6) (2000) 931–9.

Doyal, L., Cottingham, J., Garcia-Moreno, C., Hartigan, P. and Sims, J., *Gender and Health: A Technical Paper* (World Health Organisation: http://www.who.int/frh-whd/GandH/GHreport/gendertech.htm#, 1998).

Drife, J., 'Data on Babies' Safety during Hospital Births are Being Ignored', *British Medical Journal,* 319 (1999) 1008.

Dunn J. and Brown, J., 'Affect Expression in the Family, Children's Understanding of Emotions and their Interactions with Others', *Merrill-Palmer Quarterly,* 40 (1) (1994) 120–37.

Durkheim, E., *Rules of Sociological Method* (New York: Free Press, 1964 [1895]).

Ebrahim, S., 'Caring for Older People: Ethnic Elders', *British Medical Journal,* 7 (313) (1996) 610–13.

Edwards, G., 'Long Term Outcome for Patients with Drinking Problems: The Search For Predictors', *British Journal of Addiction,* 83 (1988) 917–27.

Edwards, G., *The Treatment of Drinking Problems: A Guide for the Helping Professions* (Oxford: Blackwell Publications, 1989).

Elkind, A.K., Haran, D., Eardley, A. and Spencer, B., 'Well You Can Come in but I'm Not Having it', *Health Visitor,* 62 (1989) 20–1.

Ellenwood, E.H., Smith J.P. and Vallient, G.E., 'Narcotic Addictions in Males and Females: A comparison', *International Journal of the Addictions,* 1 (2) (1966) 33–45.

Elliott, C.M., *Signs of our Times* (Basingstoke: Marshall Pickering, 1988).

Erens, B., Primatesta, P. and Prior G., *Health Survey for England: The Health of Minority Ethnic Groups 1999.* (London: The Stationery Office, 2000).

Esping-Andersen, G., *The Three Worlds of Welfare Capitalism* (Cambridge: Polity Press, 1990).

Estês, C.P., *Women Who Run With the Wolves* (London: Rider at Random House, 1992).

Ettore, B., 'Women, Substance Abuse and Self-help', in S. MacGregor, *Drugs and British Society: Responses to a Social Problem in the Eighties* (London: Routledge, 1989) 101–15.

Ettore, B., *Women and Substance Use* (Basingstoke: Macmillan, 1992).

Ettore, E. and Riska, E., *Gendered Moods* (London: Routledge, 1993).

Evans, J., *Feminist Theory Today. An Introduction to Second-wave Feminism* (London; Thousand Oaks, CA; New Delhi: Sage, 1995).

Ewles, L. and Simnett, I. *A Practical Guide to Health Promotion,* (London: Scutari, 1995).

Fairhurst, I., *Women Writing in the Person-Centred Approach* (Ross-on-Wye: PCCS Books, 1999).

Falkov, A., 'Fatal Child Abuse and Parental Psychiatric Disorder', *Part 8 Review,* (London: HMSO, 1997).

Farah, N.K., *A Continent Called Palestine: One Woman's Story* (London: Triangle, 1996).

Faris, R.E.L. and Dunham, H.W., *Mental Disorders in Urban Areas* (Chicago: University of Chicago Press, 1965 [1939]).

Fathalla, M.F., 'Fertility Control Technology: A Women-Centered Approach to Research', in G. Sen et al. (eds), *Population Policies Reconsidered: Health, Empowerment, and Rights* (Boston: Harvard University Press, 1994).

Faust, J., Runyon, M.K. and Kenny, M.C., 'Family Variables Associated with the Onset of Intra-familial Childhood Sexual Abuse', *Clinical Psychology Review,* 15 (5) (1995) 443–56.

Favazza, A. and Conterio, K., 'The Plight of Chronic Self-Mutilators', *Community Mental Health Journal,* 24 (1988) 22–30.

Favazza, A., 'Why Patients Mutilate Themselves', *Hospital and Community Psychiatry*, 40 (1989) 137–45.

Favazza, A., *Bodies under Siege: Self-Mutilation and Body Modification in Culture and Psychiatry*, 2nd edn (Baltimore: The Johns Hopkins University Press, 1996).

Ferguson, C., *Global Social Policy Principles: Human Rights and Social Justice* (London: DFID, 1999).

FIGO Committee Report, 'FIGO Committee for the Ethical Aspects of Human Reproduction and Women's Health', *International Journal of Obstetrics and Gynaecology*, 64 (1999) 317–22.

Finkelhor, D., *Sexually Victimised Children* (New York: Free Press, 1979).

Finkelhor, D., *Child Sexual Abuse: New Theory and Research* (New York: Free Press, 1984).

Finkle, J.L. and McIntosh, C.A. (eds), *The New Politics of Population: Conflict and Consensus in Family Planning* (New York: The Population Council, 1994).

Fishbein, M and Ajzen, I. *Belief, Attitude, Intention and Behaviour: An Introduction to Theory and Research* (Reading, MA: Addison-Wesley, 1975).

Flesch, R., *The Art of Readable Writing* (New York: Harper and Row, 1949).

Foucault, M., 'Governmentality', in G. Burchell, C. Gordon and P. Miller (eds), *The Foucault Effect* (Hemel Hempstead: Harvester Wheatsheaf, 1991a).

Foucault, M., *Discipline and Punish* (Harmondsworth: Penguin, 1991b).

Foucault, M., *Madness and Civilisation* (London: Tavistock, 1967).

Fox, N. *Postmodernism, Sociology and Health* (Milton Keynes: Open University Press, 1993).

Francome, C., *Changing Childbirth* (London: Maternity Alliance, 1989).

Francome, C., Savage, W., Churchill, H. and Lewison, H., *Caesarean Birth in Britain-A Book for Health Professionals and Parents* (Middlesex University Press in association with The National Childbirth Trust, 1993).

Fraser, N., *Unruly Practices: Power, Discourse and Gender in Contemporary Social Theory* (Cambridge: Polity Press, 1989).

Freedman L.P. and Isaacs, S.L., 'Human Rights and Reproductive Choice', *Studies in Family Planning*, 24 (1) (1993) 18–30.

Freeman, A., 'The Development of Treatment Conceptualisations in Cognitive Therapy', in A. Freeman and F. Detillio (eds), *Comprehensive Casebook of Cognitive Therapy* (New York: Plenum Press, 1992).

Freud, S., 'Mourning and Melancholia', in P. Rieff (ed.), *Sigmund Freud: General Psychological Theory: Papers on Metapsychology* (New York: Collier Books, 1917) pp. 164–79.

Freud, S., 'Three Essays on the Theory of Sexuality', in *Freud 7: On Sexuality* (Harmondsworth: Penguin 1977 [1905]).

Gabe, J. (ed.), *Medicine, Health and Risk* (Oxford: Blackwell, 1995).

Galaif, E.R., Nyamathi, A.M. and Stein, J.A., 'Psychosocial Predictors of Current Drug Use, Drug Problems and Physical Drug Dependence in Homeless Women', *Addictive Behaviours*, 24 (6) (1999) 801–14.

Gallagher, J., 'Prenatal Invasions and Interventions: What's Wrong with Fetal Rights?', *Harvard Women's Law Journal*, 10 (1987) 9.

Garcia, J., Kilpatrick R. and Richards, M., *The Politics of Maternity Care: Services for Childbearing Women in Twentieth-century Britain* (Oxford: Oxford University Press, 1990).

Gardner, S., *Substance Abuse during Pregnancy*, Social Work Monograph (Norwich: UEA, 1992).

Garner R. and Butler, G., 'Learning from Acts of Deliberate Self-harm', *Psychiatric Care*, Nov/ Dec (1994) 197–201.

Gendlin, E., *Focusing* (revised edn) (New York: Bantam Books, 1981).

Gendlin, E., *Focusing-Oriented Psychotherapy: A Manual of the Experiential Method* (New York: Guilford Press, 1996).

General Medical Council, *Tomorrow's Doctors* (London: GMC Press, 1993).

General Medical Council, *Duties of a Doctor* (London: GMC Press, 1995).

General Register Office, The Registrar General's Decennial Supplement, England and Wales, 1931. Part IIa, *Occupational Mortality* (London: HMSO, 1938).

George, C., 'A Representational Perspective of Child Abuse and Prevention: Internal Working Models of Attachment and Caregiving', *Child Abuse and Neglect*, 20 (5) (1996) 411–24.

Germain, A., Holmes, K., Piot, P. and Wasserheit, J., *Reproductive Tract Infections: Global Impact and Priorities for Women's Reproductive Health* (New York: Plenum Press, 1992).

Gibbons, M. and Cazottes, I. 'Working with women's Groups to Promote Health in the Community using the Health Analysis and Action Cycle within Nepal', *Qualitative Health Research*, 11 (6) (2001) 728–50.

Giddens, A., *Modernity and Self-Identity* (Cambridge: Polity Press, 1991).

Gijsbers van Wijk, C., VanVliet, K. and Kolk, A.-M., 'Gender Perspectives and Quality of Care: Towards Appropriate and Adequate Health Care for Women', *Social Science and Medicine*, 43 (5) (1996) 707–20.

Gillan, A. and Ward, L. 'Prostitutes Imported into Slavery', *The Guardian*, 30 May 2000.

Gillick, M., 'Health Promotion, Jogging and the Pursuit of the Moral Life', *Journal of Health Politics, Policy and the Law*, 9 (3) (1984) 369–87.

Ginn J. and Arber, S., 'Changing Patterns of Pension Inequality: The Shift from State to Private Sources', *Ageing and Society*, 19 (1999) 319–42.

Ginn, J and Arber, S., 'Ethnic Inequality in Later Life: Variation in Financial Circumstances by Gender and Ethnic Group', *Education and Ageing*, 15 (1) (2000) 65–83.

Ginn, J., Arber S. and Cooper, H., *Researching Older People's Health Needs and Health Promotion Issues* (London: Health Education Authority, 1997).

Glaser, B.G. and Strauss, A.L., *The Discovery of Grounded Theory* (Chicago: Adline, 1967).

Glaser, D. and Prior, V., 'Is the Term Child Protection Applicable to Emotional Abuse?', *Child Abuse Review*, 6 (1997) 315–29.

Glassner, B., *Bodies: Overcoming the Tyranny of Perfection* (Chicago: Contemporary Books, 1992).

Gloppen S. and Rakner, L., *Human Rights and Development: The Discourse in the Humanities and Social Sciences* (Bergen: CMI, 1993).

Gold, S.N., Hughes, D.M. and Swingle, J.M., 'Characteristics of Childhood Sexual Abuse among Female Survivors in Therapy', *Child Abuse and Neglect*, 20 (1996) 323–35.

Goldberg D. and Huxley, P., *Common Mental Disorders* (London: Routledge, 1992).

Goldstein, J.E., *Console and Classify: The French Psychiatric Profession in the Nineteenth Century* (Cambridge: Cambridge University Press, 1987; paperback edn, 1990; French translation, 1997).

Goldstein, J.M., 'Gender and Schizophrenia: A Summary of Findings', *Schizophrenia Monitor*, 2 (1992) 1–4.

Goldstein, M.S., *The Health Movement. Promoting Fitness in America* (New York: Twayne Press, 1992).

Goldstein, P.J., *Prostitution and Drugs* (Lexington, MA: Lexington Books, 1979).

Goodwin, S., *Comparative Mental Health Policy* (London: Sage, 1997).

Gordon J. and Barrett, K., 'The Co-dependency Movement: Issues of Context and Differentiation', in M. Baer, G.A. Marlatt and M. McMahon (eds), *Addictive Behaviours across the Lifespan: Prevention, Treatment and Policy Issues* (California: Sage, 1993).

Gove, W., 'The Relationship between Sex Roles, Marital Status and Mental Illness', *Social Forces*, 51 (1972) 34–44.

Gowdridge C. (ed.), *Mother Courage: Letters from Women in Poverty at the End of the Century* (Harmondsworth: Penguin, 1997).

Grace QC, J., 'Should the Foetus have Rights in Law?', *Medico-Legal Journal*, 67 (1999) 57.

Graham, H. and Oakley, L., 'Competing Ideologies of Reproduction: Medical and Maternal Perspectives on Pregnancy', in H. Roberts (ed.), *Women, Health and Reproduction* (London: Routledge and Kegan Paul, 1981).

Graham, W.J., Huntley, V., McCheyne, A.L., Hall, M.H., Gurney, E. and Milne, J., 'An Evaluation of Women's Involvement in the Decision to Deliver by Caesarean Section', *British Journal of Obstetrics and Gynaecology*, 106 (1999) 213–20.

Gray, C., 'Anti-Retrovirals and Their Role in Preventing Mother to Child Transmission of HIV-1' in UNAIDS (ed.) (Geneva: World Health Organisation, 1998).

Green, J., Coupland V.A. and Kitzinger, J.V., *Great Expectations: A Prospective Study of Women's Expectations and Experiences of Childbirth* (Cambridge: Child Care and Development Group, 1988).

Greenberger, D. and Padesky, C., *Mind over Mood. Change How You Feel by Changing How You Think* (New York: Guilford Press, 1996).

Greene, M.E., 'Changing Women and Avoiding Men: Gender Stereotypes and Reproductive Health Programmes', *IDS Bulletin*, 31 (2) (2000) 49–59.

Greenhalgh (ed.), S., *Situating Fertility: Anthropology and Demographic Enquiry* (Cambridge: CUP, 1995).

Greenhalgh, S., 'Fresh Winds in Beijing: Chinese Feminists Speak out on the One-Child Policy and Women's Lives', *Journal of Women in Culture and Society*, 26 (3) (2001) 847–56.

Greer, G., *The Change: Women, Ageing and the Menopause* (London: Hamish Hamilton, 1991).

Gregory, D., 'What happens to children when their parents have mental health problems?' (University of East Anglia: unpublished MA Dissertation, 1997).

Gregory-Bills, T. and Rhodeback, M., 'Comparative Psychopathology of Women who Experienced Intra-familial versus Extra-familial Sexual Abuse', *Child Abuse and Neglect*, 19 (1995) 177–89.

Greig, A. and Howe, D., 'Social Understanding, Attachment Security of Pre-School Children and Maternal Mental Health', *Journal of Developmental Psychology*, 19 (2001) 381–93.

Grinyer, A., 'Risk, the Real World and Naïve Sociology: Perceptions of Risk from Occupational Injury in the Health Service', in J. Gabe (ed.), *Medicine, Health and Risk* (Oxford: Blackwell, 1995).

Grubb, G.S., 'Human Papillomavirus and Cervical Neoplasia: Epidemiological Considerations', *International Journal of Epidemiology* 15 (1986) 1–7.

H.M. Inspectorate of Prisons, *Women in Prison in England and Wales: A Thematic Review* (London: Home Office, 1997).

Hall, M.H., 'Audit', in G. Chamberlain and N. Patel (eds), *The Future of the Maternity Services* (London: RCOG Press, 1994).

Hall, P., Ward, E., 'Cervical Screening for Women with Learning Disability: Numbers Screened can be Optimised by Using a Focused Initiative', *British Medical Journal,* 318 (1999) 536–7.

Hamilton, J., 'Women and Health Policy: On the Inclusion of Females in Clinical Trials', in C. Sargent and C. Brettell (eds), *Gender and Health: An International Perspective* (Upper Saddle River, NJ: Prentice Hall, 1996).

Hammen, B., 'Children of Affectively Ill Parents', in H.C. Steinhausen and F. Verhulst (eds), *Risks and Outcomes in Developmental Psychopathology* (Oxford: Oxford University Press, 1999) pp. 38–53.

Hammersley M. and Atkinson, P., *Ethnography: Principles in Practice* (London: Tavistock, 1983).

Hammersley, R., Forsyth A. and Lavelle, T., 'The Criminality of New Drug Users in Glasgow', *British Journal of Addiction,* 85 (1990) 1583–94.

Hancock, P., 'Rural Women Earning Income in Indonesian Factories: The Impact on Gender Relations', *Gender and Development,* 9 (1) (2001) 18–24.

Hanmer J. and Statham, D., *Women and Social Work: Towards a Woman-Centred Practice* (Basingstoke: Macmillan, 1988).

Hannah M. and Hannah, W., 'Caesarean Section or Vaginal Birth for Breech Presentation at Term. We Need Better Evidence as to which is Better', *British Medical Journal,* 312 (1996) 1433–4.

Harcourt, W., *Power, Reproduction and Gender: The Intergenerational Transfer of Knowledge* (London: Zed, 1997).

Harris, J., *The Value of Life: An Introduction to Medical Ethics* (London: Routledge, 1985).

Hausermann, J., *Rights and Humanity: A Human Rights Approach to Development, Discussion Paper* (London: DFID, 1998).

Havelock, C.M., Edwards, R., Cuzick, J. and Chamberlain, J., 'The Organisation of Cervical Screening in General Practice', *Journal College of General Practitioners,* 38 (1988) 207–11.

Havelock, C.M., Webb, J. and Queenborough, J., 'Preliminary Results of a District Call Scheme for Cervical Screening Organised in General Practice', *British Medical Journal,* 297 (1988) 1317–18.

Hawton K. and Catalan, J., *Attempted Suicide* (Oxford: Oxford University Press, 1987).

Haynes, S., 'The Effect of Job Demands, Job Control and New Technologies on the Health of Employed Women: A Review', in M. Frankenhaueser, U. Lundberg and M. Chesney (eds), *Women, Work and Health: Stress and Opportunities* (New York: Plenum Press, 1991).

Health Advisory Service, *Together We Stand* (London: HMSO, 1995).

Health Education Authority, *Black and Minority Ethnic Groups in England* (London: HEA, 1994).

Health Education Authority, *Can You Avoid Cancer?* (London: HEA, 1988).

Health Education Authority, *Health and Lifestyles: A Survey of the UK Population* (London: HEA, 1995).

Health Education Authority, *Black and Minority Ethnic Groups in England: The Second Health and Lifestyles Survey* (London: HEA, 1999).

Heise, L., Moore, K. and Toubia, N., *Sexual Coercion and Reproductive Health: A Focus on Research* (New York: Population Council, 1995).

Henderson, J. and Mugford, M., 'Economic Evaluation of Home Birth', in G.V.P. Chamberlain and A. Wraight (eds), *National Birthday Trust Fund Confidential Inquiry into Home Births* (London: Parthenon, 1997) pp. 191–211.

Henderson, S., 'Drugs and Culture: The Question of Gender', in N. South, *Drugs, Cultures and Controls in Everyday Life* (London: Sage, 1999).

Hewson, B., 'Case Analysis', *Journal of Civil Liberties*, 2 (1997) 44.

Hewson, B., 'When "No" Means "Yes" ', *Law Society Gazette*, 45 (1992) 2.

Hewson, B., 'Women's Rights and Legal Wrongs', *New Law Journal*, 146 (1996) 1385.

Hicks, A. (1996) *The Principles of Chinese Medicine* (London: Thorsons, 1996).

Hodgson, R., 'Treatment of Alcohol Problems; Section 5, Treatment', *Addiction*, 89 (1994) 1529–34.

Hogg, C., *Drug Using Parents and their Children* (London: SCODA, 1989).

Holland, J., Ramazanoglou, C., Scott, S., Sharpe, S., and Thomson, R., 'Sex, Gender and Power: Young Women's Sexuality in the Shadow of AIDS', *Sociology of Health and Illness*, 12 (3) (1990) 336–50.

Hollingshead A.B. and Redlich, F.C., *Social Class and Mental Illness* (New York: Wiley, 1958).

House of Commons Health Committee [Chair, N. Winterton], *Maternity Services: Second Report*, Session 1991–92, HC29–1, Vol. I (London: HMSO, 1991).

House of Commons Health Committee [Chair, N. Winterton], *Maternity Services: Preconceptual care, Antenatal Care and Delivery, Second Report*, Session 1991–2, Vol. II (London: HMSO, 1992).

House of Commons Social Services Committee, *Government's Reply to the Second Report on Perinatal and Neonatal Mortality* (London: HMSO, 1980).

Irion, O., Hirsbrunner Almagbaly, P. and Morabia, A., 'Planned Vaginal Delivery versus Elective Caesarean Section: A Study for 705 Singleton Term Breech Presentations', *British Journal of Obstetrics and Gynaecology*, 105 (1998) 710–17.

Jack, R.,*Women and Attempted Suicide* (Hove: Lawrence Erlbaum Associates, 1992).

Jackson, C., 'Post Poverty, Gender and Development', *IDS Bulletin*, 28 (3) (1997) 145–55.

Jackson, N.V. and Irvine, L.M., 'The Influence of Maternal Request on the Elective Caesarean Section Rate', *British Journal of Obstetrics and Gynaecology*, 18 (1998) 115–19.

Jackson, S., *Melancholia and Depression* (New Haven: Yale University Press, 1987).

Jacob, T., 'Psychosocial Functioning in Children of Alcoholic Fathers', *Journal of Studies on Alcohol*, 47 (5) (1986) 373–80.

Jacobson, J., 'Women's Health, the Price of Poverty', in M. Koblinsky, J. Timyan and J. Gay (eds), *The Health of Women: A Global Perspective* (Boulder, CO: Westview Press, 1993).

Jain A. and Bruce, J., 'A Reproductive Health Approach to the Objectives and Assessment of Family Planning Programs', in G. Sen et al. (eds), *Population Policies Reconsidered: Health, Empowerment, and Rights* (Boston: Harvard University Press, 1994).

James, J., 'Prostitution and Addiction: An Interdisciplinary Approach', *Addictive Diseases: An International Journal,* 2 (4) (1976) 601–18.

James, K., *The Depressed Mother: A Practical Guide to Treatment and Support* (London: Cassell, 1998).

Jefferies, S., 'Heroin Addiction Beyond the Stereotype', *Spare Rib* (July 1983) 6–8.

Jehu, D., *Beyond Sexual Abuse: Therapy with Women who were Childhood Victims* (Chichester: Wiley, 1988).

Johnson E. and Britt, B., *Self-Mutilation in Prisons* (Illinois: Carbondale, 1967).

Joint Committee of the Royal College of Obstetricians and Gynaecologists and the Population Investigation Committee, *Maternity in Great Britain* (London: Oxford University Press, 1948).

Jordanova, L., *Sexual Visions: Images of Gender in Science and Medicine between the 18th and 19th Centuries* (Madison: University of Wisconsin Press, 1989).

Joshi, H., Paci P. and Waldfogel, J., 'The Wages of Motherhood: Better or Worse?', *Cambridge Journal of Economics,* 23 (5), Special issue on the family (1999) 543–64.

Kabeer, N. and Cook, S., 'Editorial Introduction: Revisioning Social Policy in the South: Challenges and Concepts', *IDS Bulletin,* 31 (4) (2000) 1–10.

Kadden R. and Kranzler, H., 'Alcohol and Drug Abuse Treatment at the University of Connecticut Health Centre', *British Journal of Addiction,* 87 (4) (1992) 521–6.

Kahan, J. and Pattison E., 'Proposal for a Distinctive Diagnosis: the Deliberate Self-Harm Syndrome', *Suicide and Life Threatening Behavior,* 14 (1984) 17–35.

Kaplan A. and Surrey, J., 'The Relational Self in Women', in L. Walker (ed.), *Women and Mental Health Policy* (Beverly Hills: Sage 1984).

Keene, J., *Alcohol Treatment: A Study of Therapists and Clients* (Aldershot: Avebury, 1994).

Keene, J., *Drug Misuse. Prevention, Harm Minimisation and Treatment* (London: Chapman and Hall, 1997).

Keene, J., *Clients with Complex Needs: Interprofessional Practice* (Oxford: Blackwell Science, 2001).

Keil, T.J., 'Sex Role Variations and Women's Drinking', *Journal of Studies on Alcohol,* 39 (1978) 859–68.

Kemshall, H., *Risk in Probation Practice* (Aldershot, Brookfield, Singapore, Sydney: Ashgate, 1998).

Kent, D., 'The Negro Aged', *The Gerontologist,* 11 (1971) 48–51.

Kent, R., *Say When: Everything a Woman Needs to Know about Alcohol and Drinking Problems* (London: Sheldon Press, 1989).

Kirkham, M., 'An Evaluation of Information and Choice in Maternity Care', in *Women's Informed Childbearing and Health Services* (Report by Sheffield University, 1999).

Kitzinger, S., *Re-discovering Birth* (Boston, New York, London: Little, Brown, 2000).

Kolder V. et al., 'Court-Ordered Obstetrical Interventions', *New England Journal of Medicine,* 19 (1987) 1192.

Koopmanschap, M., van Oortmarssen, G., Van Agt, H.M. and Ballengoojen, M., 'Cervical Cancer Screening: Attendance and Cost Effectiveness', *International Journal of Cancer*, 45 (1990) 410–15.

Koss, M., 'The Women's Mental Health Research Agenda: Violence against Women', *American Psychologist*, 45 (3) (1990) 374–80.

Kovacs, M., 'The Emanuel Miller Memorial Lecture 1994 – Depressive Disorders in Childhood: An Impressionistic Landscape'. *Journal of Child Psychology and Psychiatry*, 38 (3) 287–98.

Kraepelin, E., *Psychiatrie*, 5th edn (Leipzig: Barth, 1896).

Kumar, R., 'Maternal Depression and the Emotional Development of the Child', *British Journal of Psychiatry*, 154 (1989) 818–23.

LaBarge, M.W., *A Small Sound of the Trumpet: Women in Medieval Life* (Boston: Beacon Press, 1986).

Ladwig G.B. and Anderson, M.D., 'Substance Abuse in Women: The Relationship Between Chemical Dependency of Women and Past Reports of Physical and/or Sexual Abuse', *The International Journal of the Addictions*, 24 (8) (1989) 739–54.

Lee, H., *To Kill a Mockingbird* (Harmondsworth: Penguin, 1960).

Leitner, M., Shapland J. and Wiles, P., *Drug Usage and Drug Prevention: the Views and Habits of the General Public*, Home Office Report (London: HMSO, 1993).

Lerner, M., *Surplus Powerlessness* (Englewood Cliffs, London: Humanities Press, 1991).

Ley, P., 'The Measurement of Comprehensibility', *Journal – Institute of Health*, 11 (1973) 17–20.

Lilford, R.J., 'The Relative Risks of Caesarean Section and Vaginal Delivery', *British Journal of Obstetrics and Gynaecology*, 97 (1990) 883–92.

Lindstrom, L., *Managing Alcoholism. Matching Clients to Treatments* (Oxford: Oxford University Press, 1992).

Llewelyn Davies, M. (ed.), *Maternity: Letters from Working Women*. Collected by the Women's Co-operative Guild (London: G. Bell and Sons, 1915).

Lloyd, M., 'Feminism, Aerobics and the Politics of the Body', *Body and Society*, 2 (2) (1996) 79–98.

Loudon, I., *The Tragedy of Childbed Fever* (Oxford: Oxford University Press, 2000).

Louveau, C., 'La Forme, Pas Les Formes! Simulacres et Equivoques dans le Pratique Physique Féminines', in C. Pociello (ed.), *Sport et Société* (Paris: Vigot, 1981).

Lowe, M., *Women of Steel. Female Body Builders and the Struggle for Self-Definition* (New York: New York University Press, 1998).

Lowndes, V., 'Women and Social Capital: A Comment on Hall's "Social Capital in Britain"', *British Journal of Political Science*, 30 (2000) 533–40.

Lublin, N., *Pandora's Box: Feminism Confronts Reproductive Technology* (New York: Rowman & Littlefield, 1998).

Lunbeck, E., *The Psychiatric Persuasion* (Princeton: Princeton University Press, 1994).

MacDonald, M., *Mystical Bedlam: Madness, Anxiety and Healing in Seventeenth Century England* (Cambridge: Cambridge University Press, 1981).

Macfarlane, A. and Mugford, M., *Birth Counts: Statistics of Pregnancy and Childbirth*, 2 volumes (London: HMSO, 1984).

Macfarlane, A. and Mugford, M., *Birth Counts: Statistics of Pregnancy and Childbirth* Volume 1 Text, 2nd edn (London: The Stationery Office, 2000).

Macfarlane, A., Mugford, M., Henderson, J., Furtado, A., Stevens J. and Dunn, A., *Birth Counts: Statistics of Pregnancy and Childbirth*, Volume 2 Tables, 2nd edn (London: The Stationery Office, 2000).

Macintosh, M., 'The Family in Socialist-Feminist Politics', in R. Brunt and C. Rowan (eds), *Feminism, Culture and Politics* (London: Lawrence and Wishart, 1986).

Mackenzie, I.Z., 'Should Women who Elect to have Caesarean Sections Pay for Them?', *British Medical Journal*, 318 (1999) 1070.

Maguire J. and Mansfield, L., ' "No-body's Perfect": Women, Aerobics and the Body Beautiful', *Sociology of Sport Journal*, 15 (2) (1998) 109–37.

Main, M., 'Metacognitive Knowledge, Metacognitive Monitoring and Singular vs. Multiple (Incoherent) Models of Attachment', in C. Murray Parkes, J. Stevenson-Hinde and P. Harris (eds), *Attachment across the Life Cycle* (London: Tavistock, 1991) pp. 127–59.

Malon, D. and Beradi, D., 'Hypnosis with Self-cutters', *American Journal of Psychotherapy*, 50 (4) (1987) 531–41.

Manning, N., 'Psychiatric Diagnosis under Conditions of Uncertainty: Personality Disorder, Science and Professional Legitimacy', *Sociology of Health and Illness*, 22 (2000) 621–39.

Mansfield, A. and McGinn, B., 'Pumping Irony: The Muscular and the Feminine', in S. Scott and D. Morgan (eds), *Body Matters. Essays on the Sociology of the Body* (London: The Falmer Press, 1993).

Markula, P., 'Firm but Shapely, Fit but Sexy, Strong but Thin: The Postmodern Aerobicizing Female Bodies', *Sociology of Sport Journal*, 12 (4) (1995) 424–53.

Martinson, D., Secret Shame website (1998) URL: http://palace.net/~llama/psych/selfinjury.html.

MATCH Research Group, 'Matching Alcoholism Treatments to Client Heterogeneity: Project MATCH Post-treatment Outcomes', *Journal of Studies on Alcohol*, 58 (1997).

McCormick, E.W., *Nervous Breakdown: A Positive Guide to Coping, Healing and Rebuilding* (London: Unwin, 1988).

McGuffin P. and Sargeant, M.P., 'Genetic Markers and Affective Disorder', in P. McGuffin and R. Murray (eds), *The New Genetics of Mental Illness* (Oxford: Butterworth-Heinemann, 1991) pp. 165–81.

McIlwaine, G., Cole, S. and Macnaughton, M., 'The Rising Caesarean Section Rate – A Matter for Concern', *Health Bulletin*, 43 (1985) 301–5.

McIntyre, S., 'Obstetric Routines in Antenatal Care'. Paper given at British Sociological Association Medical Sociology Group Conference at York, 1976.

McNicoll, G., 'Institutional Analysis of Fertility', in K. Lindahl-Kiessling, and H. Landberg (eds), *Population, Economic Development, and the Environment* (Oxford: OUP, 1994).

Meltzer, H., Gill, B., Petticrew, M. and Hinds, K., *The Prevalence of Psychiatric Morbidity amongst Adults Living in Private Households* (London: Office of Population Censuses and Surveys, 1995).

Meredith, B., *Foreword: Vogue Body and Beauty Book* (London: Book Club Associates, 1981).

Merton, P., Harmer, A. and Sanderson, J., 'Influence of Negative Childhood Experiences on Psychological Functioning, Social Support and Parenting for Mothers Recovering from Addiction', *Child Abuse and Neglect*, 23 (5) (1999) 421–33.

MIDIRS, Informed Choice Leaflet No. 9, 'Breech Baby – What Are Your Choices?' (MIDIRS Midwives Information and Resource Service, Bristol, 1997).

Mihill, C., 'Vaccine Hope for Cervical Cancer "Virus"', in *The Guardian*, (14 September 1990) 3.

Miles, A., *Women, Health and Medicine* (Milton Keynes: Open University Press, 1991).

Mill, J.S., *Three Essays: Medicine* (Milton Keynes: Open University Press, 1975).

Miller, D., *Women Who Hurt Themselves: A Book of Hope and Understanding* (New York: Basic Books, 1994).

Miller, P., 'Critiques of Psychiatry and Critical Sociologies of Madness', in N. Rose and P, Miller (eds), *The Power of Psychiatry* (Cambridge: Polity Press, 1987).

Millman, M. (ed.), *Access to Health Care in America* (Washington: National Academy Press, 1993).

Ministry of Health, Maternity Services Committee [Chair, Lord Cranbrook], *Report on Maternity Services* (London: HMSO, 1959).

Ministry of Health, *Memorandum with Regard to Maternity Homes and Hospitals* 15/MCW (London: HMSO, 1920).

Mintzes, B., (ed.), *A Question of Control: Women's Perspectives on the Development and Use of Contraceptive Technology* (Amsterdam: Women and Pharmaceuticals Project, Health Action International and WEMOS, 1992).

Mirsky J. and Radlett M. (eds), *No Paradise Yet: The World's Women Face the New Century* (London: PANOS/Zed, 2000).

Mitchell, J., *Psychoanalysis and Feminism* (Harmondsworth: Penguin, 1974).

Moi, T., *Sexual/Textual Politics* (London: Routledge, 1985).

Moore, H., *Feminism and Anthropology* (Oxford: Polity Press, 1988).

Moore, J. and Hawtin, S., 'Empowerment or Collusion? The Social Context of Person-Centred Therapy', in Thorne B. and Lambers, E. (eds), *Person-Centred Therapy: A European Perspective* (London: Sage, 1998).

Moorhead, J. 'Parents 2: The Panel' *The Guardian* (10 May 2000).

Moos, R.H., Finney, J.W. and Cronkite, R.C., *Alcoholism Treatment: Context, Process and Outcome* (Oxford: Oxford University Press, 1990).

Morse, M., 'Artemis Aging: Exercise and the Female Body on Video', *Discourse*, 10 (1987/1988) 19–53.

Mullen, P.E., Martin, J.L., Anderson, J.C., Romans, S.E. and Herbison, G.P., 'The Long-term Impact of the Physical, Emotional and Sexual Abuse of Children: A Community Study', *Child Abuse and Neglect*, 20 (1) (1996) 7–21.

Murray, L., 'The Impact of Postnatal Depression on Infant Development', *Journal of Child Psychology*, 33 (1992) 543–61.

Murray, L. and Trevarthen, C., 'Emotion Regulation and Interactions between Two-month-olds and Their Mothers', in T.M. Field and N.A. Fox (eds), *Social Perception in Infants* (Norwood, NJ: Ablex, 1991).

Najavits, L.M., Weiss, R.D. and Shaw, S.R., 'The Link between Drug Abuse and Post-traumatic Stress Disorder in Women: A Research Review', *American Journal on Addictions*, 6 (4) (1997) 273–83.

National Abortion Rights Action League, 'Limitations on the Rights of Pregnant Women', in *Fact Sheet on Abortion and the Law* (NARAL, 21 March 2001).

Navarro, V., *Medicine under Capitalism* (New York: Prodist, 1976).

Nazroo, J.Y., 'Ethnic Inequalities in Health', in D. Gordon et al. (eds), *Inequalities in Health* (Bristol: The Policy Press, 1999).

Nazroo, J.Y., *Ethnicity and Mental Health* (London: Policy Studies Institute, 1997a).

Nazroo, J.Y., *The Health of Britain's Ethnic Minorities* (London: Policy Studies Institute, 1997b).

Nelson-Zlupko, L., Kauffman, E. and Morrison Dore, M., 'Gender Differences in Drug Addictions and Treatment: Implications for Social Work Intervention with Substance-Abusing Women', *Social Work*, 40 (1) (1995) 45–54.

Nesse R.M. and Williams, G.C., *Evolution and Healing: The New Science of Darwinian Medicine* (London: Phoenix, 1996).

Neuberger J. and Kyle, C., *Whatever's Happening to Women?* (London: Kyle Cathie, 1991).

Newman, K. and Helzner, J.F., 'IPPF Charter on Sexual and Reproductive Rights', *Journal of Women's Health and Gender-Based Medicine*, 8 (4) (1999) 459–63.

Nightingale, C., 'Barriers to Health Access; A Study of Cervical Screening for Women with Learning Disabilities', *Clinical Psychology Forum*, 137 (March 2000) 26–30.

Nightingale, C., 'Issues of access to health services for people with learning disabilities: A case study of cervical screening' (unpublished PhD, 1997).

Norman, A., 'Triple Jeopardy: Growing Old in a Second Homeland', *Policy Studies in Ageing*, 3 (London: Centre for Policy on Ageing, 1985).

Norman-Bruce, G. and Kearney, P., '"Abusers Twice Over": An Account of a Multi-disciplinary Training Day in Child Protection for Drugs Workers', *Social Work Education*, 9 (1) (1990) 3–13.

Norris, J., Nurius, P.S. and Dimeff, L.A., 'Through Her Eyes: Factors Affecting Women's Perceptions of and Resistance to Acquaintance Sexual Aggression Threat', *Psychology of Women Quarterly*, 20 (1996) 132–45.

Northam, S., 'Access to Health Promotion, Protection and Disease Prevention among Impoverished Individuals', *Public Health Nursing*, 13 (5) (1996) 353–64.

Norton, A., 'Can There be a Global Standard for Social Policy? The Social Policy Principles as a Test Case', Overseas Development Institute Briefing Paper No. 2, (London: ODI, 2000).

Oakley, A., *Subject Women* (Oxford: Martin Robertson; New York: Pantheon Books, 1981).

Oakley, A., *The Captured Womb: A History of the Medical Care of Pregnant Women* (Oxford: Blackwell, 1984).

Oberman, M., 'Real and Perceived Legal Barriers to the Inclusion of Women in Clinical Trials', in A. Dan (ed.), *Reforming Women's Health: Multidisciplinary Research and Practice* (London: Sage, 1996).

Obermeyer, C.M., 'A Cross Cultural Perspective on Reproductive Rights', *Human Rights Quarterly*, 17 (1995) 366–81.

Office for National Statistics (ONS) *Social Trends*, 30 (London: The Stationery Office, 2000).

Office for National Statistics (ONS), Series DH3 No. 31 *Mortality Statistics: Childhood, Infant and Perinatal for England and Wales* (London: ONS, 1998).

Office for Population Censuses and Surveys, *Mortality Statistics: Childhood, Infant and Perinatal for England and Wales* (London: OPCS, 1995).

Oja, P. and Tuxworth, B., *Eurofit for Adults. Assessment of Health-Related Fitness* (Tampere: Council of Europe, 1995).

Oliver, S., 'Users of Health Services: Following their Agenda', in S. Hood, B. Mayall and S. Oliver (eds), *Critical Issues in Social Research: Power and Prejudice* (Buckingham: Open University Press, 1999).

Oppenheim, J., *Shattered Nerves* (New York: Oxford University Press, 1991).

Oppenheimer, E., 'Women Drug Misusers: A Case for Special Consideration', in J. Strang and M. Gossop, *Heroin Addiction and Drug Policy: the British System* (Oxford: Oxford University Press, 1994).

Orford J. and Vellman, R., 'Offspring of Parents with Drinking Problems', *British Journal of Addiction*, 85 (1996) 779–94.

Oxley, W.H.F., Phillips, M.H. and Young, J., 'Maternal Mortality in Rochdale', *British Medical Journal*, 1 (1935) 304–7.

Padesky, C.A. and Greenberger, D., *Clinician's Guide to Mind over Mood* (New York: Guilford Press, 1995).

Padesky, C.A., 'Schema Change Processes in Cognitive Therapy', *Clinical Psychology and Psychotherapy*, 1 (5) (1994) 267–78.

Palmer, S., *Introduction to Counselling and Psychotherapy: The Essential Guide* (London: Sage, 2000).

Palmore, E. and Manton, K., 'Ageism Compared to Racism and Sexism', *Journal of Gerontology*, 28 (3) (1973) 363–9.

Paltrow, L.M., 'Pregnant Drug Users, Fetal Persons, and the Threat to *Roe* v *Wade*', *Albany Law Review*, 63 (1999) 999.

Park, R.J., 'A Decade of the Body: Researching and Writing about the History of Health, Fitness, Exercise and Sport, 1983–1993', *Journal of Sport History*, 21 (1) (1994) 59–82.

Patel, N., 'Healthy Margins: Black Elders' Care – Models, Policies and Prospects', in W.I.U. Ahmad (ed.), *'Race' and Health in Contemporary Britain* (Buckingham: Open University Press, 1993).

Paterson-Brown S. and Fisk, N.M., 'Caesarean Section: Every Woman's Right to Choose?', *Current Opinion in Obstetrics and Gynaecology*, 9 (1999) 351–5.

Pavalko, E.K. and Woodbury, S., 'Social Roles as Process: Caregiving Careers and Women's Health', *Journal of Health and Social Behaviour*, 41 (1) (2000) 91–105.

Pearson, R. and Seyfang, G., 'New Hope or False Dawn? Voluntary Codes of Conduct, Labour Regulation and Social Policy in a Globalising World', *Global Social Policy*, 1 (1) (2001) 77–106.

Pearson, V., Davis, C., Ruoff, C. and Dyer, J., 'Only One Quarter of Women with Learning Disability in Exeter have Cervical Screening', *British Medical Journal*, 316 (1998) 1979.

Pembroke, L. (ed.), *Self-Harm: Perspectives from Personal Experience* (London: Survivors Speak Out, 1994).

Persons, J.B., *Cognitive Therapy in Practice: A Case Formulation Approach* (New York: W.W. Norton, 1989).

Petchesky, R.P. and Judd, K. (eds), *Negotiating Reproductive Rights: Women's Perspective across Countries and Cultures* (London: Zed, 1998).

Petchesky, R.P., *Reproductive and Sexual Rights* (UNRISD Occasional Paper No. 8: Geneva, 2000).

Phelan, J.B., 'The Maternal Abdominal Wall: A Fortress against Fetal Health Care?', *Southern California Law Review*, 65 (1991) 461.

Phipps, C., 'Just Take Two Aspirin and Call Us Next Century', *The Guardian* (21 December 1999) 8.

Pierce, M., Lundy, S., Palenisimmy, A., Winning, S. and King, J., 'Prospective Randomised Controlled Trial of Methods of Call and Recall for Cervical Cytology Screening', *British Medical Journal*, 299 (1989) 160–2.

Plant, M., *Women and Alcohol: A Review of the International Literature on Use of Alcohol by Females* (Geneva: World Health Organisation, 1990).

Plaut, G., 'My Practice Screening Audit Shows High Cancer Incidence', *Pulse*, 46(2) (11 January 1986) 47.

Plichta, S.B.,'Violence and Abuse: Implications for Women's Health', in M.M. Falik and K.S. Collins (eds), *Women's Health: The Commonwealth Fund Survey* (Baltimore: Johns Hopkins University Press, 1996).

Poland, F., 'Trading Relationships: Home Selling and Petty Enterprise in Women's Lives', in S. Arber and N. Gilbert (eds), *Women and Working Lives: Divisions and Change* (London: Macmillan, 1991).

Presser, H.B. and Sen, G. (eds), *Women's Empowerment and Demographic Processes: Moving beyond Cairo* (Oxford: Oxford University Press, 2000).

Priest, J., *Drugs in Pregnancy and Childbirth* (London: Pandora, 1990).

Prior, P., *Gender and Mental Health* (London: Macmillan, 1999).

Prochaska, J.O. and DiClemente, C.C. 'Transtheoretical Therapy toward a More Integrative Model of Change', *Psychotherapy: Theory Research and Practice* (1982).

Putnam, R., 'The Prosperous Community: Social Capital and Public Life', *American Prospect*, 13 (1993) 35–42.

Quinn, S., 'Woman Whose Smear Test was Forgotten Dies', *The Guardian*, (23 January 1999) 11.

Rabinbach, A., *The Human Motor. Energy, Fatigue, and the Origins of Modernity* (New York: Basic Books, 1990).

Rader, B.J., 'The Quest for Self-Sufficiency and the New Strenuosity', *Journal of Sport History*, 18 (2) (1991) 255–76.

Radke-Yarrow, M., McCann, K., DeMulder, E., Belmont, B., Martinez, P. and Richardson, D.T., 'Attachment in the Context of High Risk Conditions', *Development and Psychopathology*, 7 (1995) 247–65.

Ramirez, F.O. and McEneaney, E.H., 'From Women's Suffrage to Reproductive Rights? Cross-National Considerations', *International Journal of Comparative Sociology*, 38 (1997) 6-24.

Ramon, S., 'The Category of Psychopathy: Its Professional and Social Context in Britain', in N. Rose and P. Miller (eds), *The Power of Psychiatry* (Cambridge: Polity Press, 1987).

Rana, R., Smith, E. and Walkling, J., 'Degrees of Disturbance: The New Agenda – The Impact of Increasing Levels of Psychological Disturbance amongst Students in Higher Education'. Report produced by the Heads of University Counselling Services Forum (1999).

Rawcliffe, C., *Medicine and Society in Later Medieval England* (Stroud: Sutton Publishing, 1995).

Reichenheim, M. and Harpham, T., 'Maternal Mental Health in a Squatter Settlement in Rio de Janeiro', *British Journal of Psychiatry* 159 (1991) 683–90.

Reinharz, S., *Feminist Methods in Social Research* (Oxford: Oxford University Press, 1992).

Richards, J.R., *The Sceptical Feminist: A Philosophical* Enquiry (London: Penguin, 1994).

Roberts, D.E., 'Punishing Drug Addicts Who have Babies: Women of Color, Equality, and the Right of Privacy', *Harvard Law Review*, 104 (1991) 1419.

Roberts, H. (ed.), *Women, Health and Reproduction* (London: Routledge, 1981).

Robinson, J., *On the Demon Drink* (London: Mitchell Beazley, 1988).

Rocheron, Y., 'The Asian Mother and Baby Campaign: The Construction of Ethnic Minority Health Needs', *Critical Social Policy*, 22 (1988) 4–23.

Rogers, C., *Client-Centered Therapy* (London: Constable, 1951).

Rosenbaum, M., *Women on Heroin* (New Brunswick, NJ: Rutgers University Press, 1981).

Rosenberg , H., 'The Home is the Workplace: Hazards, Stress and Pollutants in the Household', in W. Chavkin (ed.), *Double Exposure: Women's Health Hazards on the Job and at Home* (New York: Monthly Review Press, 1984).

Rosenfeld, Q., Nadelson, C., Krieger, M. and Backman, J., 'Incest and Sexual Abuse of Children', *Journal of the American Academy of Child Psychiatry*, 16 (1979) 327–39.

Rosenstock, I.M., Strecher, V.J. and Becker, M.H., 'Social Learning Theory and the Health Belief Model', *Health Education Quarterly*, 15 (2) (1988) 175–83.

Ross, S.K., 'Cervical Cytology Screening and Government Policy', *British Medical Journal*, 299 (1989) 101–4.

Rosser, S., 'Gender Bias in Clinical Research: The Difference it Makes', in A. Dan (ed.), *Reforming Women's Health: Multidisciplinary Research and Practice* (London: Sage Publications, 1994).

Ross-Gower, J., Waller, G., Tyson, M. and Elliot, P., 'Reported Sexual Abuse and Subsequent Psychopathology among Women Attending Psychology Clinics: The Mediating Role of Dissociation', *British Journal of Clinical Psychology*, 37 (1998) 313–26.

Rowland, R., *Living Laboratories: Women and Reproductive Technology* (Bloomington: Indiana University Press, 1992).

Roy, R., 'Consequences of Parental Illness in Children', *Social Work and Social Sciences Review*, 2 (2) (1991) 109–21.

Royal College of Obstetricians and Gynaecologists, 'Response to Winterton Report', (London: British Journal of Obstetrics and Gynaecology Press, 1992) p. 4, para 5.

Royal College of Obstetricians and Gynaecologists, *Recommendations to the Future of Maternity Services* (London: Royal College of Obstetricians and Gynaecologists Press, 1993).

Russell, D., *The Secret Trauma: Incest in the Lives of Girls and Women* (New York. Basic Books, 1986).

Russell, H., 'Friends in Low Places: Gender, Unemployment and Sociability', *Work, Employment and Society*, 13 (1999) 205–24.

Salasin, S.E. and Rich, R.E., 'Mental Health Policy for Victims of Violence: The Case against Women', in J. Wilson and B. Raphael (eds), *International Handbook of Traumatic Stress Syndromes* (New York; London: Plenum Press, 1993).

Sassatelli, R., 'Interaction Order and Beyond. A Field Analysis of Body Culture within Fitness Gyms', *Body and Society*, 5 (2–3) (1999a) 227–48.

Sassatelli, R.,'The Gym and the Local Organization of Experience', *Sociological Research Online*, 4 (3) (1999b) www.socresonline.org.uk/.

Sassatelli, R., *Anatomia della Palestra e Cultura Commerciale* (Bologna: il Mulino, 2000).

Savage, W., *A Savage Enquiry* (London: Virago Press, 1986).

Savage, W. and Francome, C., 'British Caesarean Section Rates: Have We Reached a Plateau?', *British Journal of Obstetrics and Gynaecology*, 100 (1993) 493–6.

Savage, W., Schwartz, M. and George, J., *A Study of Women's Knowledge, Attitudes, and Experience of Cervical Screening in the Tower Hamlets Health District* (London: The Medical College of St Bartholomew's Hospital, 1989).

Schaef, A.W., *Escape from Intimacy* (New York: HarperCollins, 1989).

Scheff, T.J., *Being Mentally Ill: A Sociological Theory*, 3rd edn (New York: de Gruyter, 1999 [1967]).

Schneidman, E. and Faberow, N., *The Cry for Help* (New York: McGraw-Hill, 1961).

Schutz, A., *On Phenomenology and Social Relations*, edited and introduction by H.R. Wagner (Chicago, London: University of Chicago Press, 1970).

Schwartz, A. and Schwartz, R.M., *Depression: Theories and Treatments. Psychological, Biological and Social Perspectives* (New York; Oxford: Columbia University Press, 1993).

SCODA, *Drug Using Parents: Policy Guidelines for Interagency Working* (London: LGA Publications, 1997).

Scott, S and Freeman, R. 'Prevention as a Problem of Modernity,' in J. Gabe (ed.), *Medicine, Health and Risk* (Oxford: Blackwell, 1995).

Scottish Home and Health Department, *Provision of Maternity Services in Scotland. A Policy Review* (Edinburgh: HMSO, 1993).

Scull, A., 'From Madness to Mental Illness: Medical Men as Moral Entrepreneurs', *Archives Européenes de Sociologie*, 16 (1975) 218–61.

Scull, A., *Decarceration: Community Treatment, A Radical View* (Englewood Cliffs: Prentice Hall, 1977).

Scull, A., *Museums of Madness* (London: Allen Lane, 1979).

Seligman, L.E.P., 'Depression and Learned Helplessness', in R.J. Friedman and M.M. Katz (eds), *The Psychology of Depression: Contemporary Theory and Research* (Washington: Winston, 1974).

Sen, A., 'Family and Food: Sex Bias in Poverty', in T. Srinivasan and P. Bardham (eds), *Rural Poverty in South Asia* (New York: Columbia University Press, 1988).

Sen, A., 'Gender and Cooperative Conflicts', in I. Tinker (ed.), *Persistent Inequalities: Women and World Development* (Oxford: OUP, 1990).

Sen, G., Germain, A. and Chen, L., *Population Policies Reconsidered: Health, Empowerment and Rights* (Boston, Harvard University Press, 1994).

Sen, G. and Snow, C.R. (eds), *Power and Decision: The Social Control of Reproduction* (Boston: Harvard University Press, 1994).

Shearer, A., *Woman: Her Changing Image: A Kaleidoscope of Five Decades* (Wellingborough: Thorsons, 1987).

Shephard, R.J., 'Physical Activity, Fitness and Health. The Current Consensus', *Quest*, 47 (3) (1995) 288-303.

Sheppard, M., 'Social Work, General Practice and Mental Health Sections: The Social Control of Women', *British Journal of Social Work*, 21 (1991) 663–83.

Short Report, *Perinatal and Neonatal Mortality. Second Report from the Social Services Committee, Session 1979–80* (London: HMSO, 1980).

Showalter, E., *The Female Malady: Women, Madness and English Culture 1830–1981* (London: Virago, 1987).

Shuttleworth, S., 'Female Circulation: Medical Discourse and Popular Advertising in the mid-Victorian Era', in M. Jacobus, E.F. Keller and S. Shuttleworth (eds), *Body/Politics* (London: Routledge, 1990).

SID (The Society for International Development), *Development*, 42 (1) (1999).

Singer, A. and Yule, R., 'Cervical Cancer Hits Younger Women', *General Practitioner*, (28 September 1984) 3.

Skinner, B.F., *Science and Human Behaviour* (New York: The Free Press, 1953).

Small Group, *Report on Suicide among Rural Chinese Women* (Guiyang: Guizhou People's Press, 1999).

Smith, A. and Jackson, B. (eds), *The Nation's Health: A Strategy for th 1990s* (London: King Edward's Hospital Fund for London, 1988).

Smith, D., 'The Statistics on Mental Illness: What They Will Not Tell Us about Women and Why', in D.E. Smith and S.J. David (eds), *Women Look at Psychiatry* (Vancouver: Press Gang, 1975).

Smith, G., Cox, D. and Saradjian, J., *Women and Self-Harm* (London: The Woman's Press, 1998).

Smith, P., *The Emotional Labour of Nursing* (Basingstoke: Macmillan, 1992).

Smith, R., *Trial by Medicine: Insanity and Responsibility in Victorian Trials* (Edinburgh: Edinburgh University Press, 1981).

Smith-Rosenberg, C., 'Puberty to Menopause: The Cycle of Femininity in Nineteenth-century America', in M. Harmann and L.W. Banner (eds), *Clio's Consciousness Raised* (New York: Harper and Row, 1974).

Solomon, H.A., *The Exercise Myth* (New York: Harcourt, 1984).

Sontag, S., *Illness as Metaphor* (New York: Penguin, 1978).

Stacey, M., *The Sociology of Health and Healing* (London: Routledge, 1988).

Stainton Rogers, W. *Explaining Health and Illness* Hemel Hempstead: Harvester/Wheatsheaf, 1991.

Standing Maternity and Midwifery Advisory Committee [Chair, J. Peel], *Domiciliary Midwifery and Maternity Bed Needs* (London: HMSO, 1970).

Standing, H., 'Gender and Equity in Health Sector Reform Programmes: A Review', *Health Policy and Planning*, 12 (1) (1997) 1–18.

Staunton, P., 'The Rise of the Modern Urban Shaman', *Prediction* (May 2000) 25–31.

Stein, K. and Allen, N., 'Cross-sectional Survey of Cervical Cancer Screening in Women with Learning Disability', *British Medical Journal*, 318 (1999) 641.

Stengal, E., *Suicide and Attempted Suicide* (Harmondsworth: Penguin, 1964).

Stewart, T., *The Heroin Users* (London: Pandora, 1987).

Strang, J. and Gossop, M., *Heroin Addiction and Drug Policy: The British System* (Oxford: Oxford University Press, 1994).

Strauss A. and Corbin, J., *Basics of Qualitative Research: Techniques and Procedures for Developing Grounded Theory*, 2nd edn (London: Sage, 1998).

Sullivan, W.P. and Hartmann, D.J., 'Implementing Case Management in Alcohol and Drug Treatment', *Families in Society*, 75 (2) (1994) 67–73.

Sullivan, W.P., Wolk, J.L. and Hartmann, D.J., 'Case Management in Alcohol and Drug Treatment: Improving Client Outcomes', *Families in Society*, 73 (1992) 195–204.

Sultan, A. and Stanton, S., 'Preserving the Pelvic Floor and Perineum-elective CS?', *British Journal of Obstetrics and Gynaecology*, 103 (1996) 731–4.

Surrey, J., Swett, C., Michaels, A. and Levin, S., 'Reported History of Physical and Sexual Abuse and Severity of Symptomatology in Women Psychiatric Outpatients', *American Journal of Orthopsychiatry*, 60 (1990) 412–17.

Tantam, D. and Whittaker, J., 'Personality Disorder and Self-Wounding', *British Journal of Psychiatry*, 161 (1992) 451–64.

Task Force, *Caesarean Childbirth* (Washington, DC: US Institute of Health and Human Services, 1981).

Taylor, A., *Women Drug Users: An Ethnography of a Female Drug Using Community* (New York: Clarendon Press, 1994).

Tew, M., *Safer Childbirth? A Critical History of Maternity Care* (London, New York: Chapman and Hall, 1990).

Thaddeus, S. and Maine, D., *Too Far to Walk: Maternal Mortality in Context* (New York: Centre for Population and Family Health, Faculty of Medicine, Columbia University, 1991).

Thom, B. and Green, A., 'Services for Women; The Way Forward', in L. Harrison (ed.) *Alcohol Problems in the Community* (London: Routledge, 1996).

Thorne, B., *Carl Rogers* (London: Sage, 1992).

Thornton, J.G. and Lilford, R.J., 'The Caesarean Section Decision: Patients' Choices are not Determined by their Immediate Emotional Reactions', *Journal of Obstetrics and Gynaecology* 9 (1989) 283–8.

Timyan, J., Brechin, S., Measham, D. and Ogunleye, B., 'Access to Care: More than a Problem of Distance', in M. Koblinsky, J. Timyan and J. Gay, *The Health of Women: A Global Perspective* (Boulder CO: Westview Press, 1993).

Tones, K. J. And Tilford, S. *Health Promotion: Effectiveness, Efficiency and Equity* (London: Nelson Thomas. 2001).

Tong, R., *Feminist Thought: A Comprehensive Introduction* (London: Unwin Hyman, 1989).

Toth, R.L. and Cicchetti, D., 'Patterns of Relatedness, Depressive Symptomatology, and Perceived Competence in Maltreated Children', *Journal of Consulting and Clinical Psychology*, 64 (1) (1996) 32–41.

Toubia, N. and Izett, S., *Female Genital Mutilation: An Overview* (Geneva: World Health Organisation, 1998).

Townsend, P. and Davidson, N., *Inequalities in Health: The Black Report* (London: Penguin, 1988).

Tracey, E.M. and Farkas, K.J., 'Preparing Practitioners for a Child Welfare Practice with Substance-abusing Families', *Child Welfare,* 73 (1) (1994) 57–68.

Treffers, P.E., Eskes, M., Kleiverda, G. and van Alten, D., 'Home Births and Minimal Medical Intervention', *JAMA,* 264 (1990) 2203–8.

Turner, B.S.,*The Body and Society* (London: Sage, 1984, 2nd edn, 1996).

UN (United Nations), *Copenhagen Declaration on Social Development and Programme of Action of the World Summit for Social Development,* (UN Doc A/Conf. 166/9, 1995).

UN (United Nations), *Programme of Action of the International Conference on Population and Development* (UN Doc A/Conf.171/13, 1994).

UNAIDS, *Update on the HIV/AIDS Epidemic* (Geneva: World Health Organisation, 1998).

United Nations, 'The World's Women 1970–1990: Trends and Statistics', *Social Statistics and Indicators,* Series K 12 (New York: UN, 1995).

Ussher, J. *Women's Madness: Misogyny or Mental Illness* (London: Harvester Wheatsheaf, 1991).

Ussher, J.M. and Dewberry, C., 'The Nature and Long-term Effects of Childhood Sexual Abuse: A Survey of Adult Women Survivors in Britain', *British Journal of Clinical Psychology*, 34 (1995) 177–92.

Vaz , K.M. (ed.), *Oral Narrative Research with Black Women* (Thousand Oaks, CA: Sage, 1997).

Vigarello, G., *Le Corps redressé: Histoire d'un pouvoir pédagogique* (Paris: Delarge, 1978).

Wagner, M., *Pursuing the Birth Machine* (Camperdown, NSW: Ace Graphics, 1994).

Waites, B., 'Into the Breech. A Consumer's Point of View', *The Practising Midwife*, 2 (1) (1999) 30–4.

Waldron, I. and Jacobs, J., 'Effects of Labor Force Participation on Women's Health: New Evidence from a Longitudinal Study', *Journal of Occupational Medicine*, 30 (12) (1989) 977–83.

Walker, M., *Women in Therapy and Counselling* (Milton Keynes: Open University Press, 1990).

Warner, R., *Recovery from Schizophrenia*, 2nd edn (London: Routledge, 1994).

Waterson, E.J. and Ettore, B., 'Providing Services for Women with Difficulties with Alcohol or Other Drugs', *Drug and Alcohol Dependence*, 24 (1989) 119–25.

Weeks, M., Singer, M., Grier, M. and Schensul, J., 'Gender Relations, Sexuality and AIDS Risk among African American and Latina Women', in C. Sargent and C. Brettell (eds), *Gender and Health: An International Perspective* (Upper Saddle River, NJ: Prentice Hall, 1996).

Weisberg, D.K., *Children of the Night: A Study of Adolescent Prostitution* (Lexington, MA: Lexington Books, 1985).

Weismann, M.M. and Klerman, G.L., 'Gender and Depression', *Trends in Neuroscience*, 8 (9) (1985) 416–20.

Welsh Health Planning Forum, *Protocol for Investment in Health Gain: Maternal and Early Child Health* (Cardiff: NHS Directorate, 1992).

Werner, D. (1995) 'The Village Health Worker: Lackey or Liberator?' in B. Davey, A. Gray, and C. Seale (eds.) *Health and Disease: A Reader* (Buckingham: Open University Press).

West J. and Pilgrim, S., 'South Asian Women in Employment: The Impact of Migration, Ethnic Origin and the Local Economy', *New Community*, 21 (3) (1995) 357–78.

West, C. and Zimmerman, D.H., 'Doing Gender', *Gender and Society*, 1 (2) (1987) 125–51.

White, P., Young, K. and Gillett, J., 'Bodywork as a Moral Imperative. Some Critical Notes on Health and Fitness', *Loisir et Société*, 18 (1) (1995) 159–81.

Whiteside, A. and Sunter, C., *AIDS: The Challenge for South Africa* (Cape Town: Human and Rousseau Tafelberg, 2000).

Whitmore, J., 'Cervical Screening for Women with Learning Disability: Sefton has Multidisciplinary Group to Promote Sexual Health Care for these Women', *British Medical Journal*, 318 (1999) 537.

Whitty, N., 'The Mind, the Body and Reproductive Health Information', *Human Rights Quarterly*, 18 (1996) 224–39.

Wilkinson, C., McIlwaine, G., Boulton-Jones, C. and Cole, S., 'Is a Rising Caesarean Section Rate Inevitable?', *British Journal of Obstetrics and Gynaecology*, 105 (1998) 45–52.

Wilkinson, R.G., *Unhealthy Societies. The Afflictions of Inequality* (London: Routledge, 1996).

Williams, A.S., *Women and Childbirth in the twentieth century: A History of the National Birthday Trust Fund, 1928–93* (Stroud: Sutton, 1997).

Williamson, V., 'Users First: From Policy to Practice' in V. Williamson (ed.), *Users First. The Real Challenge for Community Care* (Brighton: University of Brighton, 1993).

Winnicott, D., *Home is Where We Start From* (Harmondsworth: Penguin, 1986).

Winnicott, D., *Playing and Reality* (London: Hogarth, 1971).

Winnicott, D., *The Child, the Family and the Outside World* (Harmondsworth: Penguin, 1964).

Winschel, R.M. and Stanley, M., 'Self-Injurious Behaviour: A Review of the Behaviour and Biology of Self-mutilation', *American Journal of Psychiatry*, 148 (30) (1991) 306–15.

Wolf, N., *Fire with Fire* (London: Vintage, 1994).

Wolfson, D. and Murray, J. (eds), *Women and Dependency* (London: Dawn, 1986).

Woodhouse, D. and Pengelley, P., *Anxiety and the Dynamics of Collaboration* (Aberdeen: Aberdeen University Press, 1991).

Wootton, B., *Social Science and Social Pathology* (London: Allen and Unwin, 1959).

World Bank, *World Development Indicators* (Geneva: World Bank, 1998).

World Health Organisation, Expert Committee on Drug Dependence, 28th Report, (Geneva: World Health Organisation, 1989).

World Health Organisation, *Why Do Mothers Suffer and Die?* (Geneva: Safe Motherhood Newsletter, Issue 1 (6–7), WHO, Division of Family Health, 1989).

World Health Organisation, *The ICD-10 Classification of Mental and Behavioural Disorders* (Geneva: World Health Organisation, 1992).

World Health Organization, *International Statistical Classification of Diseases and Related Health Problems*, 10th Revision (Geneva: World Health Organization, 1994).

World Health Organisation, *Women, Ageing and Health: Achieving Health across the Life Span* (Geneva: World Health Organisation, 1996).

World Health Organisation, *Women's Health: Improve Our Health, Improve our World* [WHO Position Paper, Fourth World Conference on Women] (Geneva: World Health Organisation, WHO/FHE/95.9, 1995).

Yates, A., *Compulsive Exercise and Eating Disorders. Toward an Integrated Theory of Activity* (New York: Brunner/Mazel, 1991).

Yin, R.K., *Case Study Research: Design and Methods* (Beverly Hills: Sage, 1989).

Young, J.E., *Schema-focused Cognitive Therapy for Personality Disorders: A Schema Focused Approach* (Saratoga, FL: Professional Resource Exchange, 1990).

Zahn-Waxler, C., Kochanska, G., Krupruk, J. and McKnew, D., 'Patterns of Guilt in Children of Depressed and Well Mothers', *Developmental Psychology*, 26 (1) (1990) 51–9.

Zimmer-Hofler, D. and Nikla-Mikola, A., 'Swiss Heroin-addicted Females: Career and Social Adjustment', *Journal of Substance Abuse Treatment*, 9 (1992) 159–70.

Name Index

Nelson-Zlupko, M., Kauffman, G. and
　Dore, A., 69–70, 72–3, 75
Nesse, R.M. and Williams, G.C., 22
Neuberger, J. and Kyle, C., 31
Newman, K. and Helzner, R.F., 215
Nightingale, C., 15, 156–7, 220
Norman, A., 72, 194
Norman-Bruce, G. and Kearney, P., 72
Norris, J., Nurius, P.S. and Dimeff,
　L.A., 5
Northam, S., 156
Norton, A., 219

Oaker, G., 9, 15, 129
Oakley, A., 108, 173
Obermeyer, C.M., 213–14
Oja, P. and Tuxworth, B., 77, 82
Oliver, S., 190
OPCS, 65
Oppenheim, J., 37, 44
Oppenheimer, E., 66–7, 69, 75
Orford, J. and Vellman, R., 65
Oxley, W.H.F., Philips, M.H. and
　Young, J., 184

Padesky, C.A., 131, 140, 143
Padesky, C.A. and Greenberger, D.,
　140
Palmer, S., 90
Palmore, E. and Manton, K., 194
Paltrow, L.M., 117, 119
Park, R.J., 81, 88
Patel, N., 195
Paterson-Brown, S. and Fisk, N.M.,
　110
Pavalko, E.K. and Woodbury, S., 156
Pearson, V., Davis, C., Ruoff, C. and
　Dyer, J., 159
Pearson, R. and Seyfang, S., 218
Pembroke, L., 52–6, 59, 61–4
Persons, J.B., 130
Petchesky, R.P., 209, 213–17, 220
Petchesky, R.P. and Judd, K., 208,
　210–11, 214
Phipps, C., 156
Pierce, M., Lundy, S., Palenisimmy,
　A., Winning, S. and King, J., 158
Plant, M., 66–7, 70, 76
Plaut, G., 158

Plichta, S.B., 5
Poland, F., 1, 13
Priest, J., 65
Prochaska, J.O. and DiClemente,
　C.C., 16
Putnam, R., 12

Quinn, S., 159

Rabinbach, A., 81
Rader, B.J., 86
Radke-Yarrow, M., McCann, K.,
　DeMulder, E., Belmont, B.,
　Martinez, P. and Richardson,
　D.T., 149
Ramirez, F.O. and McEneaney, E.H.,
　211–12, 215
Ramon, S., 45
Rana, R., Smith, E. and Walkling, J.,
　90
Rawcliffe, C., 23–4, 35
Reichenheim, M. and Harpham, T., 9
Reinharz, S., 55, 59
Roberts, H., 108
Robinson, J., 66, 70
Rocheron, Y., 195
Rogers, C., 91–2, 97, 99–100
Rosenbaum, M., 67, 70–1
Rosenfeld, Q., Nadelson, C., Krieger,
　M. and Backman, J., 129
Rosenstock, I.M., Strecher, V.J. and
　Becker, M.H., 17
Ross, S.K., 158, 168
Rosser, S., 2
Ross-Gower, J., Waller, G., Tyson, M.
　and Elliot, P., 129
Royal College of Obstetricians and
　Gynaecologists, (RCOG), 103,
　106–7, 111, 175
Russell, D., 129
Russell, H., 12

Salasin, S.E. and Rich, R.E., 4
Sassatelli, R., 14, 77, 79, 87
Savage, W., 8, 14, 103–4, 168, 181,
　220
Savage, W. and Francome, C., 112
Savage, W., Schwartz, M. and George,
　J., 159

Subject Index